The Bump, Birth & Baby Bible

The Bump, Birth & Baby Bible

A midwife's guide through your labour of love

Lesley Gilchrist DipHb DipHE BSc (Hons) PgDip RM MHbA

Bespoke Birthing Midwifery Practice
www.bespokebirthing.co.uk

First published in Great Britain by:
Bespoke Birthing Publications, 43 Valley Drive, Harrogate, HG2 0JH

British Library Cataloguing in Publication Data
A catalogue record for this book is available from the British Library

ISBN 978-0-9930360-0-2

Editor: Mark Lister
Cover by Paula Beaumont Photography (www.paulabeaumontphotography.co.uk)
Cover artwork & design by Corvus Graphics (www.corvusgraphics.co.uk)
Illustrations by Sam West

Printed and bound in the UK by:
Printdomain.net

The information provided in this book is designed to inform you of situations that may occur in labour and afterwards and prepare you for that eventuality. It is in no way designed to replace advice or information given to you by your healthcare provider especially as situations in labour can change quickly. If you are concerned in anyway regarding your pregnancy you should contact your midwife or obstetrician for advice.

To my family,

The reason I wrote this book

CONTENTS

Part III   Parenthood

Further Information

References
Acknowledgements

INTRODUCTION

This book was written to inform women of the amazing journey of labour and birth. There are so many wonderful books on the spiritual journey of birth, but very few on the facts and decisions and fewer still from the perspective of a midwife. I felt mums to be needed the views of someone who has seen the despair of women and their partners when labour begins to take a different path, one for which they were not prepared.

The sad fact is the despair wasn't caused by changes to the birth plan or the pain or intervention in labour. It was caused by fear and anxiety felt when faced with something for which they were unprepared and at the most vulnerable point in their life. What should have been a joyful, uplifting and inspiring experience was dreadful.

The purpose of this book is to better prepare expectant mums and concerned dads to be. There is no elixir buried deep within these pages promising pain free childbirth. What this book does offer are the facts; not frightening but enlightening facts. As you will discover, anxiety and stress are the enemies of a natural labour. Fear of the unknown and fear of pain are powerful stress builders. This book will inform you, relieve you and empower you. What's more it will be a constant companion in labour for your partner, as a source of information and advice. Ultimately it will ensure that you are prepared for your birth and meet it with excitement and wonder.

Part 1

Preparing for Birth

"Nothing in life is to be feared, only to be understood."

Marie Curie (1867-1934)

Chapter 1

What is Normal Birth?

Purely by definition a normal birth is one in which a baby is born without assistance by forceps, ventouse or Caesarean section.

A natural birth is one where a woman gives birth with no assistance whatsoever from drugs for pain relief or to aid delivery of the placenta, and has no instruments to assist the birth.

When you watch popular television programmes of women giving birth you will notice that the vast majority of these women are undergoing a medicalised birth. They are using drugs for pain relief, and will tend to be lying on their backs and giving birth in bed. Were it not for the medical profession, and I include midwives in that, socialising women to accept the bed to give birth in they would feel far more accepting of using upright positions for labour and birth.

Historically, giving birth is something that women are really quite good at, experts you could say. In fact, the human race has depended on that fact; were women merely average at it we may not be here now. With this in mind why do women routinely question their ability to give birth? Is it for historical reasons or is it because medicine has brain washed women into believing that birth, a safe one, can only be achieved with their specialist knowledge and care? For some women, very few, that may be true but for most women, they give birth naturally in spite of medicine's well-meaning care.

How to Achieve This

This reluctance to perform in front of an audience is one of the reasons why most animals will find a dark secluded spot when their labour begins. It ensures that during labour they are safe and secure and to prevent predators from taking advantage of their situation. If a predator was to stumble upon them in labour, their bodies, as at any time of stress and fear would pump out adrenalin and cortisol, the 'fight or flight' or stress hormones.

These hormones act by suppressing the production of oxytocin, the labour hormone, to allow it to subside for long enough to flee to safety. It also sends blood to the muscles to aid strength in the 'fight or flight' and enable the heart to beat more effectively. Humans are no different and in our primitive form we also required that ability to flee from danger, in labour or not. That 'fight or flight' drive exists today but we recognise it as feelings of anxiety and fear. It stands to reason then that the more relaxing and calming your environment is in labour the less adrenalin and other stress hormones will be produced.

Natural selection has ensured that as a species we have survived for hundreds of thousands of years and you could argue that as time goes on we perfect the process. However, during this process of evolution, when we became less apelike, our skulls particularly our foreheads became larger to accommodate larger brains. As we evolved the front part of our brains, the neo-cortex, grew much larger. This part of our brain is where we think, problem solve and rationalise our behaviour. It's also the part that helps us to control unacceptable behaviour. With the neo-cortex accounting for two thirds of our entire brain it's the part that we use most of the time. The other part, the primitive side is used instinctively such as for breathing, eating, drinking, sleeping, sexual activity and the process of giving birth

In animals during labour the smaller neo-cortex is not used and the instinctive side of the brain takes over. However, because humans are rational thinking animals, it is almost impossible for us to consciously shut down our neo-cortex and legitimate worries and concerns intrude during labour.

Women worry about the pain they are in, the length of time they are labour and imagine what could be going wrong. The neo-cortex overrides the instinctive part of the human brain thus making the labour and birth more difficult. This thinking and resultant anxiety increases the levels of stress hormones in the body and that suppresses the production of the much needed labour hormone. If women could switch off their modern brains and revert to the primitive areas they would be able to give birth as easily as their early ancestors, and that is how hypnobirthing works.

The gradual increase in babies' head size has corresponded to an increase in the width of the female pelvis.
It would seem the greatest barrier to giving birth more easily is our front brain, so what can we do? How do we 'switch it off'? The answer is any form of relaxation, be it aromatherapy, hypnobirthing, massage and a calm and relaxed birth partner.

There is no point spending all your time trying to remain in a relaxed hypnotic state only to find your birth partner's high level of anxiety invading your serene state of mind.

Hypnobirthing

Birth hypnosis can be so effective that midwives and birth partners will be unaware that you are even in labour. Its aim is relaxation, meditation and visualisation through self-hypnosis. You would meet with a hypnobirthing teacher for a set time over a few weeks, maybe in groups or in private depending on your preference. The teacher, with the aid of CD's and books, will teach you self-hypnosis.

Women who use this talk of pain free births and immense feelings of wellbeing. Some practitioners may even support you in person through your birth if needed. As teachers will vary in the way they deliver their classes they will also differ so far as the stage of your pregnancy in which to start the course. You will ideally want to start your courses as early as possible, in your late second trimester and early third trimester to get the most benefits. For those women who start the course later in their pregnancy, provided they practise the techniques they can be just as effective at using the techniques in labour.

Breathing & Relaxation

It is all well and good to establish your need to remain as relaxed as possible throughout labour, but the problem is that the onset of labour is the time when you are most likely to become stressed and anxious. When this happens you will begin to tense your shoulders, clench your fists, your breathing will become shallow and rapid and you may begin to panic. The tensing of muscles unnecessary for the birthing process diverts important oxygen and nutrients from the placenta and uterus and the shallow and rapid breathing further reduces the amount of oxygen your body can absorb.

Relaxation can take many forms. Some women will take a course in hypnobirthing whilst others will use pregnancy yoga. Alternatively, you can try visualisation, breathing techniques and massage. Try closing your eyes for a moment. Focus on your breathing and notice how rhythmical it is. You breathe in, then there's a slight pause before you breathe out. Your out-breath matches your in-breath in length and depth, and you pause slightly before breathing in again. It is important to keep your breathing rhythmical. Try counting 'one, two, three' slowly on the breath in and 'one, two, three' slowly on the breath out. When you are having very strong contractions your breathing will become shallow. There's nothing wrong with this, but your partner can calmly talk you through this breathing technique to encourage a relaxed breathing pattern.

If you or your partner feels that your shoulders are tense then a gentle massage will help. Your partner should sit or stand behind you. Using gentle strokes they should massage down from the top of your head over your shoulder and down your back. Each single massage stroke should be timed with a breath and your partner should be gently reminding you to relax your shoulders and circle your neck.

Now I want you to imagine if you will, giving birth two hundred thousand years ago. We were extremely primitive beings then with no midwives, drugs or medical aid. Birth then was treated as a natural process and women would have been left in the company of other women or alone during that time. As this was a community the other women would ensure that her birth environment was safe from predators. It would be more likely that her labour would start during the night, similar to nowadays as at that time there would be fewer predators around. She would manage her pain in similar ways to what we do now by changing position and having her back rubbed. Then, at some point she would feel an overwhelming urge to open her bowels and would squat down to open them. She would feel a sensation similar to constipation and push harder and then all of a sudden would be unable to stop herself from pushing. Eventually her baby is born safely onto the ground.

Nowadays, the modern day obstetric experience compounds problems. Women are expected to lie slightly recumbent on a bed perhaps in lithotomy position and to give birth there. It is the most comfortable and convenient position for the midwife or obstetrician to assist you to give birth. However, there is nothing natural or instinctive about that position and it stands to reason that you are more likely to encounter problems with your labour and birth by using this position.

Positions for Labour

There are few instances in labour where you will be unable to move freely to find the position which is most comfortable for you. The only glaring exception to this would be if you were using an epidural for pain relief. The fact that you will feel less pain when using upright positions for labour is one of the strongest reasons for encouraging you to remain upright and mobile during labour. Another is that as animals we have evolved to give birth in as safe a way as possible to ensure survival of our species. As modern humans we have been socialised to fear birth and accept its medicalisation. The reason we so freely accept this medicalisation is that we have also been conditioned to feel guilt, to acquiesce to authority and to conform to social norms.

Rather than accepting the role that society expects us to play we should be playing the role that nature intended. When you are in labour you should ask yourself why certain positions feel more instinctive and natural and lying down increased the pain? To fully understand this we must go back in time to examine the fundamentals of birth.

All mammals give birth on all fours. They have the ability to lie down as they do to sleep but in labour they will instinctively find somewhere dark and secluded and remain upright. As the birth becomes imminent they will drop their hind legs in an effort to bear down reminiscent of the way we would squat to bear down. The purpose of this in human evolution is to increase the space within the pelvis in order to allow the baby's head to pass through.

In order to negotiate the different shape of your pelvis your baby's head needs to turn as he moves down which is aided by the sloping gutter shape of your pelvic floor muscles. Your pelvis is not uniformly smooth on the inside. At the back of it where the bottom of your spine joins your pelvis there is an area that protrudes known as the sacral promontory. While you are standing, the top of your pelvis is not uniformly horizontal it is tipped forwards making the angle of descent for your baby no longer straight down.

This is easily demonstrated by using a tumble drier ventilation tube, and a tennis ball. By curving the tubing upwards slightly at one end and dropping in the tennis ball it will lodge midway through the tubing. This is the same position your pelvis would be in when lying on your back requiring more effort to push your baby downwards and give birth
(Fig 1).

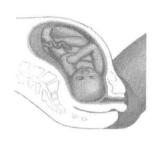
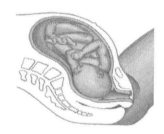
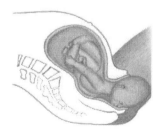
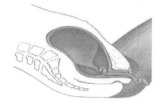

Fig 1: Baby, in the more common (occipito-anterior) spine facing position negotiating birth whilst mother lying on her back – note that the baby has to travel upwards in order to be born.

Now try holding the tubing vertically and dropping the tennis ball. This is the position your pelvis is in using an upright position. *(Fig 2)*

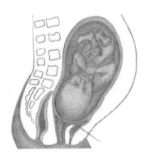
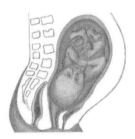
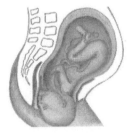
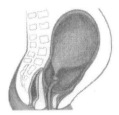

Fig 2: Baby in the normal (occipito-anterior) position negotiating birth whilst mother in an upright position – note that the baby has a simpler, downward route to be born.

If your baby is facing your back and you are leaning forward then baby is able to negotiate the passage through the birth canal easily as you have managed to change the angle at which your contractions are pushing him through your pelvis. Now imagine that he is in the same position but that you are lying down. You no longer have the gravitational force being directed through your baby's bottom forcing his head directly onto your cervix. You now have that force exerting pressure through him onto your back. The force of the contractions will still exert pressure from your baby's head onto your cervix but you are no longer using gravity to aid this. Finally, the angle at which he has to negotiate your pelvis has now changed. Rather than being able to head straight down to be born he now has to move down and backwards towards the bed and this is where the sacral promontory can cause an obstruction.

Now imagine your baby is back to back and you are lying in bed. The lack of gravitational force onto your cervix is the same but because your baby is back to back the angle at which he is trying to enter your pelvis is encouraging his head to tip further backwards. This is known as 'deflexing' and causes the diameter of your baby's head to increase. Rather than his head being tucked in where his chin can neatly fit into the space underneath it, it now sticks out. If you measure the distance from a baby's chin to the top of the back of his head (deflexed) you would expect it to measure around eleven to twelve centimetres. The measurement, the distance from his forehead to the bottom of his skull, in a tucked position will be around nine to ten centimetres.

Because the diameter of a baby's head in a back to back position is larger, it is important to either change his position so he faces your back or change your position to increase the size of your pelvis. There are a number of ways to do this, however the most effective method is either to use of a birthing stool or the toilet. If your baby is being monitored by a heart rate trace you can ask that they move the machine outside the toilet to allow you free movement

If your baby remains back to back during this period of your labour you will find most of your pain concentrated in your back. There is very little that will directly help with the pain in your abdomen but backache can be eased with massage, pressure and heat. Therefore, don't despair of a back to back labour. Remember, once your baby turns around you will feel amazing relief from the backache and benefit from the high levels of endorphins in your system. Using either a birthing stool or toilet will speed up this process.

If you remain in bed the same problems exist for you with a baby facing your back. This is due to the backwards angle that your baby will still be required to negotiate. In order to pass down through your pelvis he will exert pressure on the area of your pelvis that is in his way, your sacrum. This pressure will cause the same backache as a baby who is back to back. If you have to lie down for any period of time the best position to be in is on your left side. You will naturally curl forwards into a version of the foetal position and that way you reduce the angle of your pelvis.

Some labour wards and midwifery led units will have active birth equipment and your midwife will encourage you to use this. If there is none available there are other methods you can use with the help and support of your birth partner or midwife.

The Squat

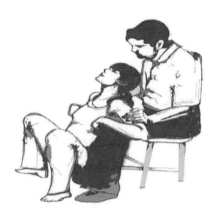

This position has a number of variations; the Western squat is the one you would use at the gym where your knees are bent at a ninety degree angle. This does not offer the maximum effect for widening your pelvis. The most effective squat is the position prevalent in the Indian Sub-continent where your vagina, rather than facing the ground faces forwards. This is not a position that Western women use frequently and because of this, even with support, you may find it difficult to maintain it for any length of time. If you have two birth partners you can use their support on either side to help you into a deep squat

The Modified Squat or Sitting

Although this position is less effective than the deep squat it has the advantage that you can maintain this position for longer especially if you use a birthing stool. If you do not have a birthing stool you can use a low stool or chair providing your knees are at the same level or higher than your hips.

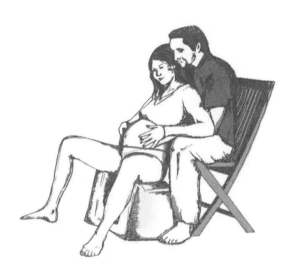

All Fours & Kneeling

If you find that you are suffering from backache then this is usually the position that will relieve it. It is a comfortable position to be in, encourages your body to lean forwards and uses the effect of gravity to aid descent of your baby. You can either use a beanbag or birthing ball to lean against or raise the back of your bed and lean over that. Most beds can be taken apart and you can ask your midwife to lower the bed down and remove the bottom of it. You will then be left with a metal shelf and a small mattress. Discard the metal shelf and place the mattress in the void on the floor and kneel onto it leaning into the crescent shape of the bed.

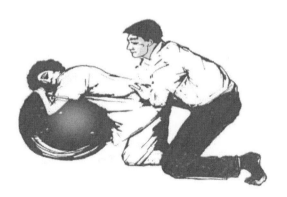

Standing

This is the easiest position to get into but again may leave you tired. You can either use your birth partner for support or lean over the bed at its full height.

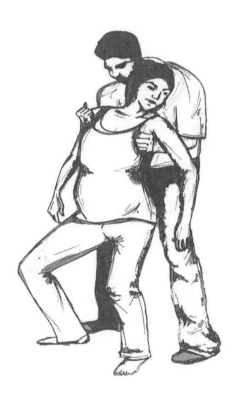

The theory behind these positions is that they all play a part in encouraging your baby to take the easiest path through your pelvis. It may be that for part of your labour he needs you in a different position and your body will instinctively know which one that is.

Don't be tempted to move positions unless it is your body telling you or your contractions have reduced. The most important message here is that labour and birth are something that as animals we will instinctively do but as humans we have become socialised to question. Hundreds of thousands of years of evolution should be your default method, banish all negative thoughts and trust your body, it will not let you down.

Your Pelvis

The type of birth that you have is largely dependent on the type of pelvis you have and there are four types; gynaecoid, platypelloid, android and anthropoid. As humans, when we moved onto our feet and become bi-peds our pelves became narrower making birth more difficult as our babies needed to negotiate a smaller pelvis. Around fifty percent of women will have a gynaecoid pelvis and these women will tend to labour in the textbook way with a baby facing your back. Twenty percent of women will have an android pelvis and those with this type of pelvis usually have a baby in the back to back position. It is most closely related to the male pelvis and this labour is characterised by back ache and a protracted labour but usually ends with a normal birth.

The platypelloid pelvis is the rarest with only around five percent of women having such. These labours are characterised by slow progress and the baby remaining sideways or occipito transverse. This pelvis and the position that your baby's head is required to move into make it the most likely to require assistance for delivery. The last pelvis type is the anthropoid and it is the most 'roomy' of all. Even if your baby is back to back, and he most likely will be, there is room for him to be born facing upwards or 'face to pubes'. These labours are usually quick, uncomplicated and most common in tall slim women.

No matter what type of pelvis you have, the most important point to remember is that nature will almost always only grow a baby to a size that your pelvis can accommodate. If you are becoming fearful of labour because everyone is telling you that you are having a big baby, relax. It means you probably just have a large pelvis. Nature seems to always find a way. So, if you are healthy with no concerns around your pregnancy then there should be no reason why you won't achieve a normal or even a natural birth.

Chapter 2

What is Pain?

Everyone's perception of pain differs. Some women find period pains agony whereas others experience them pain free. However, even those women who are cursed with severe period pains will cope. They may need to use simple pain relief such as paracetamol and hot water bottles but they cope none the less. For a woman to be incapacitated for the length of their period every month is extremely rare. Labour is no different. For a few it will be relatively quick, straightforward and require little more than water to relieve the pain, if at all. For the majority it will last for around twelve to twenty four hours and start with a gentle introduction to the sensation of the contractions. As labour progresses and the contractions become more frequent the sensation of them becomes different.

But this is not pain in the traditional sense. It is not a warning of impending danger or a nudge to seek medical advice. This time of your life is an awakening and, like being roused from sleep your body takes on a new meaning. It has grown and nourished a baby ready to be born and now is working to help you to give birth. This is not an illness or a warning of disease or something you need to be saved from.

This is a journey and the contractions that your body is having should be seen as that.

The word 'contraction' is a medical term used to describe exactly what the muscles in your uterus are doing. But labour and birth are so much more refined than that and to talk of the process of your baby being born in such simplistic medical terms is to do it an injustice. These are 'contractions' or 'rushes', as your body awakens to a new role and, with each contraction your body and your baby work in harmony. Contractions themselves are not painful. The act of the muscles in your uterus contracting and shortening to push your baby out is the same as any muscle when worked hard and it causes pain until you stop using that muscle because of the build-up of lactic acid.

When we exercise or train hard our muscles will become sore due to a lack of oxygen. If necessary we can stop and allow that pain to settle or we can push ourselves knowing that there is a benefit to this short lived pain. This is pain like any other muscle that is working hard but because it is exercise we accept that we can stop and recover if we need to. That is the natural effect of exercise. We do not decide beforehand to take pain relief in order to train harder, we embrace it. We embrace the good that it does, the way it makes us feel but most of all, we do not fear it.

Why then do we treat labour so differently? Is it because we are in that situation for longer; but what of 'ultra-runners' and 'Iron Men'? They will push their bodies for over twenty four hours, how do they manage it? The answer is that they are mentally prepared. They accept that there will be pain

29

that they will cope with it and find a way of ignoring it but they do not fear it.

That is how you should approach labour. You will not be 'having' contractions, they will be contractions of your uterus that bring your baby closer to you. The pain that you may have is just the muscles of your uterus contracting and they do this for sixty seconds on average. With each contraction you will focus on your breathing, aware that when the contraction stops the pain will cease. You are in control, this is your body and you are not a passenger. Like exercise you are asking your body to work hard for one minute and then rest, there is nothing to fear.

And essentially that is it, your body will very rarely have you in more pain than you can cope with otherwise you would be incapable of exercise or functioning through your period. You may find that you would like something to ease it and that is usually due to society and the medical profession making us believe that we need pain relief for child birth. If we are told something often enough we tend to believe it.

Pain is a very personal thing, no one will be able to understand the type of pain you have and how it makes you feel. This is true of all pain, whether you have broken your leg or are in labour. The difference with labour pain is that it has a slow build up which allows your body to produce its own pain killers to help you cope. To fully understand why we have this pain we need to understand what causes it and why.

There are three types of nerves in our bodies, motor, sensory and a mix of motor and sensory. The nerves that give us our perception of pain in labour are sensory nerves and they are found throughout our bodies. It is these nerves that pick up all the information from our uterus, our back and down through the birth canal. When doing any type of physical activity your muscles become sore and you take a rest. Muscles become sore because not enough oxygen is getting to them. If you practiced this same exercise, over time your body would become more efficient at delivering more oxygen to these muscles and you could work for longer before you felt the same pain.

Your uterus is no different. It is a large muscle, working extremely hard for days, not just hours or minutes so it stands to reason that you would experience pain from this. With any other muscle you would have stopped using it to rest it or trained your body over time to provide it with extra oxygen to work longer. With your uterus this is not possible but you can use relaxation exercises to increase the amount of oxygen that you take into your body with each breath.

I want you to imagine that you are in pain now, what does your breathing do? It speeds up and becomes shallow, limiting the amount of oxygen you take in. When you are in labour the pain is caused due to lack of oxygen to the uterus and is similar to the pain people experience during heart attacks. With a heart attack extra oxygen is given via a face mask, in labour you can simply use the breathing and relaxation exercises discussed previously. These exercises need to be reinforced by your birth partner constantly talking you through your breathing.

The other perceptions of pain you may have are the muscles of your birth canal and cervix stretching to accommodate your baby. Again breathing exercises will help with this type of pain but so will supporting yourself in water. Water is amazing for pain relief, the warmth relaxes and soothes muscles and the buoyancy ensures that the large leg muscles aren't using up too much of your body's oxygen. Just make sure the water is no hotter than thirty seven degrees centigrade otherwise the heat may cause your body to unnecessarily divert blood to your hands and feet and less to your uterus. Also, the back pain you may experience in labour may be soothed with water and breathing exercises.

For those of you experiencing a back to back labour you may experience more intense back pain rather than stomach pain and in this case it is caused by the pressure of your baby's head stretching your spine and its ligaments. The simplest way to combat this type of pain is through back massage; your partner can help here. Back rubs are very effective at relieving the severe backache associated with some positions your baby may be in. If you imagine that your baby is trying to make more room in your pelvis then it stands to reason that the bones in your pelvis that can move will move. It is the stretching of the ligaments and muscles of this bone that cause the pain. Your partner's back rub will help to take some of the pressure off and don't worry; it will not harm your baby. Here's how to do it:

Back Rub

Sit down facing the back of a chair and lean forwards.

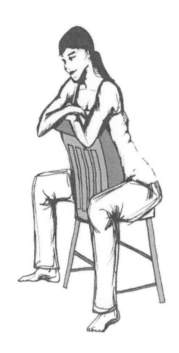

Just above the crease of your bottom your partner will see a diamond shape.

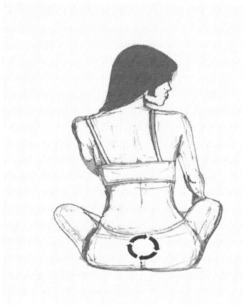

1. Ask them to put their thumbs either side of the diamond.
2. When you have a contraction ask your partner to press firmly with both thumbs until the contraction has stopped.
3. They can also use the heel of their hand on the same area.

Occasionally women find it increases their pain. If this is the case ask your partner to stop and use a heat pack or hot water bottle instead.

You also have the option of using a Transcutaneous Electrical Nerve Stimulation (TENS) machine. It works by interfering with the pain message from the sensory nerves through your spine to your brain. TENS creates a warm, buzzy sensation on your back and you can safely use it at any time in your pregnancy and labour - just remember to remove it before getting into the bath.

There is an old midwives' and nurses' saying that 'pain is what the patient says it is'; in other words, if you can feel pain and need pain relief, no matter what stage of labour you are in your midwife will accept that and provide you with what you need. However, that maxim can be a problem. As midwives we have spent years ensuring women receive pain relief when they want it, regardless of the stage of labour they are in. If you come into hospital in the early stages of labour complaining of pain your midwife may offer you strong pain relief that you cannot get at home, in the mistaken belief that you have already exhausted milder forms of pain relief.

On the other hand, if your cervix is still one centimetre dilated after two days of contractions and you are no longer coping at home, do not shy away from calling the hospital and midwife and requesting pain relief.

Chapter 3

Diet & Exercise

Strangely enough, your baby is essentially a parasite, and for any parasite to survive their host must provide them with all of their nutritional needs. Goriness aside, it is vitally important during your pregnancy to eat healthily and exercise moderately; no small task considering how unwell you may feel in the first few weeks.

Vitamins, Minerals & Supplements

Vitamins are an essential part of any diet and none more so than when you are pregnant. In order to help your body and baby during your pregnancy it is advisable to take certain vitamin supplements.

Folic Acid

The most important of these is folic acid, a form of vitamin B_9 which is found in most green leafy vegetables, brown rice and breakfast cereals fortified with vitamins and minerals. Folic acid is important for the closure of neural tubes; a deficiency in the closure of these tubes leads to spina bifida and other brain and spinal malformations.

The neural tubes however close by day 28 of the embryos life therefore it is important to begin taking folic acid before you become pregnant and preferable when you begin trying for a baby, in order to minimise your risk of these neural tube defects. The normal dosage of folic acid before conception and during pregnancy is 400 micrograms per day, and this should be continued until at least 12 weeks of pregnancy but can safely be taken throughout your pregnancy.

For some women there is an increased risk of neural tube defects, for which you will be prescribed a higher dose of 5milligrams of folic acid per day, and these include:

- If you have diabetes
- If you or your partner have a family history of neural tube defects
- If you or your partner have a neural tube defect
- If you have had a previous pregnancy affected by a neural tube defect

If you are on anti-epileptic medication you should also consult your G.P. or midwife to discuss a possible need for a higher dose of folic acid.

Vitamin D

We all need vitamin D in order to keep our teeth and bones healthy. This is especially important during pregnancy to ensure your baby has enough vitamin D for their first few months of life. A lack of vitamin D puts you at risk of rickets which leads to malformation of bones.

The best source of vitamin D is through sunshine, and 20 minutes per day of sunshine on your hands and face 3 to 4 times per week is sufficient. During the winter months this may not be possible, especially during inclement weather, and other sources of vitamin D will be required, especially if you are darker skinned or cover your skin for cultural reasons.

Good sources of vitamin D are eggs, meat and oily fish (such as salmon and mackerel) although salmon should be limited to one large tin or steak per week. As vitamin D is so important for healthy bone development in your baby some hospitals advise pregnant women to take a vitamin D supplement of 10 micrograms per day throughout their pregnancy and whilst breastfeeding.

Iron

Normal healthy iron levels are also important in pregnancy to prevent anaemia. Iron is important for red blood cell production and if you become deficient in iron you may feel tired and dizzy. Iron supplements do have side effects such as constipation and because of this it is wise to ensure that you receive adequate iron from your diet to prevent anaemia.

Lean meat, green leafy vegetables, dried fruits and nuts all contain good sources of iron and providing that you do not have a nut allergy, peanuts can be eaten as part of a balanced diet in pregnancy.

If you do suffer from tiredness and dizziness during your pregnancy do mention this to your midwife or doctor in order that they can investigate this further and offer you treatment and further diet advice.

Calcium

Your baby needs calcium in order for them to grow strong, healthy bones. By eating a diet rich in calcium you can provide your baby with all the calcium they need. Dairy products, fish with edible bones; such as sardines, breakfast cereals, dried fruits, bread, almonds, tofu, and green leafy vegetables are all good sources of calcium

Vitamin C

Your body requires vitamin C to protect the cells in your body and keep them healthy. The following fruits and vegetables contain a good source of vitamin C:

- Bell Peppers
- Blackcurrants
- Broccoli
- Citrus Fruits
- Tomatoes

What to Eat & How Much

So you know what types of food to eat, but how much of it? Well, you certainly don't need to eat for two, an extra 200 calories per day, that's an approximate total of 2200 calories per day, is quite sufficient, especially if you are eating a varied diet of fresh fruit and vegetables, pulses, fish, lean meats and proteins, nuts, seeds, fats and oils and carbohydrates.

Carbohydrates can be calorie laden so avoid white processed carbohydrates such as refined sugar, white bread, pasta, rice and peeled potatoes. Instead feast on brown bread, rice and pasta and use sweet potatoes instead of white potatoes. Refined sugar is a different matter altogether, if you can, completely eliminate it from your diet it's best to do so.

The reason that processed carbohydrates are so problematic is the effect they have on your blood sugar, creating spikes and then inevitable drops in blood sugar. This rise and fall in your blood sugars creates a craving for high carbohydrate and sugary food creating a cycle of unhealthy eating. If you can stop the cycle by introducing brown, unprocessed carbohydrates and eliminate sugar then you prevent the sugar merry-go-round, and with it the empty calories you consume.

For those women who have a raised body mass index, that is over 30, you are advised not to diet but you are encouraged to eat a healthy balanced diet within the recommended calorie intake.

Keeping Hydrated

As a general rule you should be drinking at least 1.5 litres of non-alcoholic, non-caffeinated drinks per day to avoid becoming dehydrated. If it is a particularly hot day or you've been exercising, then increase your fluid intake accordingly.

If you become dehydrated you will most likely suffer from headaches, feel dizzy and lightheaded and probably have a lower than normal blood pressure and a faster than normal pulse. If you have felt dizzy and have had headaches then please mention this to your midwife or doctor sooner rather than later as these can be symptoms of pre-eclampsia.

Diet & Anaemia

If you do become anaemic then do try to alter your diet by increasing your intake of red meat, green leafy vegetables and nuts. You can also help your body absorb the iron in these foods by drinking orange juice or any other acidic juice with meals and completely eliminate caffeine from your diet, as caffeine disrupts iron absorption.

Foods to Avoid

As much as there are many foods to eat in pregnancy, there are also many to be avoided, and for good reason. The following will explain this in more details

Liver	High vitamin A content
Non-pasteurised foods (milk, soft cheese)	Can lead to food poisoning
Mould ripened soft cheeses (brie, camembert etc.)	Can lead to food poisoning
Limit intake of oily fish (salmon, trout, tuna etc.) to 2 portions per week	Levels of pollutants found in these fish
Shark, swordfish and marlin	Avoid in pregnancy
Raw, cured and undercooked meats, fish and shellfish	Potential risk of toxoplasmosis
Alcohol	No safe limit has been determined

Soft or raw eggs (mayonnaise, carbonara)	Can lead to food poisoning
Pate	Can lead to food poisoning
Caffeine	May cause miscarriage and low birth weight babies. Limit to 2 mugs of coffee per day
Unpasteurised yoghurt	Can lead to food poisoning

What is Safe in Pregnancy

Jarred mayonnaise that uses pasteurised eggs is fine along with carbonara made without raw eggs. If you are eating fruits and vegetables make sure they are thoroughly cleaned of soil. Smoked salmon and smoked trout are considered safe to eat in pregnancy, as is shellfish, provided it is well cooked White fish are also safe to eat in pregnancy and there is no need to limit their amount. Soft, mould ripened cheeses (those with white rinds) are only safe in pregnancy if they have been thoroughly cooked. All hard cheeses such as cheddar, parmesan and stilton are considered safe in pregnancy. Yoghurt made with pasteurised milk is safe along with bio, live and low-fat varieties.

The following soft cheeses are also safe to eat in pregnancy provided they are made from pasteurised milk:

- Cottage cheese
- Mozzarella
- Feta
- Cream cheese
- Paneer
- Ricotta

- Halloumi
- Goat's cheese
- Processed cheeses such as cheese spreads

Exercise in Pregnancy

Exercise is an important part of your daily life. It helps to keep our heart and bones healthy and also our mind. In fact, some studies have shown that exercise is as effective as medication in treating depression.

Providing your pre-pregnancy exercise regime didn't involve contact sports, scuba diving, horse riding, skiing or other sports where there is potential to receive a blow to your abdomen, you can continue with this exercise. You should avoid running and other high impact exercise during pregnancy as the effects of the hormone relaxin and your baby using your pelvic floor as a trampoline do contribute to pelvic floor damage and resultant urinary incontinence.

Pilates is an excellent form of exercise for pregnancy. It builds core strength in your back, abdominal muscles and pelvic floor thereby reducing back and pelvic pain in pregnancy. For those of you who develop back or pelvic pain during pregnancy Pilates is an extremely beneficial exercise to use. Pilates also prepares you mentally for childbirth by focusing on breathing and relaxation too.

Aquanatal exercise is an excellent exercise to keep you cardiovascularly fit and also reduces the risk of pelvic floor damage brought on by high impact exercise, in fact a combination of Pilates and aquanatal exercise in pregnancy is excellent.

Pelvic Floor Exercises

Pelvic floor exercises are also vital in pregnancy and should be encouraged 3 to 4 times per week. In order to do pelvic floor exercises you need nothing more than time to do them. Doing them lying down is easiest and standing the most challenging. First of all tighten your back passage, vagina and imagine that you are trying to stop yourself from passing urine. You now should have all 3 passages squeezed, but without clenching your buttock cheeks. Now slowly lift your pelvic floor upwards towards your stomach and hold there for 10 seconds and then gently lower your pelvic floor and relax the squeeze. Now do this 10 times, 3 times per day, 3 to 4 times per week.

In no time you will notice the difference, especially during sex and your ability to hold urine and wind. You will also notice the difference during labour as a strong pelvic floor helps your baby to turn and be born.

A good rule of thumb with any exercise, and especially true in pregnancy is listen to your body, if you feel tired, stiff or in pain, stop and reassess your exercise programme; better still contact a personal trainer who specialises in prenatal exercise.

Chapter 4

Minor Ailments

Nausea & Vomiting

This usually subsides after around 16 weeks of pregnancy however ginger, keeping well hydrated, the use of antihistamines and acupressure using wrist bands may all help alleviate the symptoms. You should also avoid fatty food and eat small regular meals; little and often is the key. If you do find that you are unable to tolerate any food or fluid then you should contact your doctor or midwife for a full assessment of your condition

Varicose Veins

Sometimes they are an inevitable part of pregnancy however you can reduce their appearance, and in some cases limit their development by doing the following:

- Elevate your legs when you are able
- Take regular exercise
- Circle your ankles if you are sitting for long periods
- Consider using support stockings
- Avoid excessive weight gain

- Avoid tight waistbands and belts

Constipation

There can be a number of causes of this, namely using iron supplements and dehydration. Ensuring that you eat a diet rich in iron and fibre, especially fruit and vegetables, and increasing your fluid intake should ease the symptoms. You should avoid straining, however if the symptoms do persist you may need a gentle laxative to help things along.

Itching

Most itching in pregnancy has no treatment, only management of the itching. You can safely use calamine lotion and do try to wear loose cotton clothing and avoid scratching. In extreme cases your midwife or doctor may prescribe antihistamines for the itching. If you notice itching in the palms of your hands or soles of your feet it's important to mention this to your midwife or doctor straightaway as these could be symptoms of a condition known as obstetric cholestasis.

Haemorrhoids

This condition is usually related to straining with constipation so try the techniques to alleviate constipation and avoid straining. You can safely use topical ointments for haemorrhoids during pregnancy.

Bleeding Gums & Gingivitis

Good dental care is important during pregnancy to prevent gum disease, so brush and floss your teeth at least twice a day and visit your dentist regularly. Your midwife will have completed a form during your booking appointment, called a maternity exemption certificate which will entitle you to free prescriptions and dental treatment during your pregnancy and for one year after your baby's birth. If you have not received your maternity exemption card by the time you reach 16 weeks of pregnancy then remind your midwife of this.

Heartburn

Heartburn in pregnancy is caused by the muscle connecting your stomach to your food pipe, or oesophagus relaxing, allowing stomach acid to leak into your oesophagus. It is this acid that causes the pain. You can limit heartburn by avoiding high fat meals, spicy foods, coffee, alcohol, smoking and chocolate. You may find that you can manage the symptoms by eating small, regular meals, drinking milk and sleeping propped up on pillows. If none of these techniques work then antacids, such as gaviscon are safe to take in pregnancy, as are different medications which can be prescribed by your midwife or doctor if your heartburn is severe.

Vaginal Discharge & Thrush

It is completely normal to have an increase in vaginal discharge during your pregnancy providing it is clear, white or cream and has no accompanying itching, offensive smell or soreness. If you do notice any of these symptoms then do mention this to your midwife or doctor and they may take some samples of the discharge to test and also may prescribe ointments or antibiotics. By maintaining good levels of hygiene, wiping from front to back after using the toilet, wearing cotton underwear and avoiding tight fitting clothing such as tights and jeans, you should be able to limit these infections.

Chapter 5

Getting Organised

Where to Give Birth

The debate over the safety of homebirths has raged for some time now and increased with the Government's move in the 1970's to encourage women to give birth in hospital rather than at home. At the time it was thought that this would be the safest and cheapest place to have your baby. However, during the intervening years, medicine has increasingly tried to control a part of nature that we still know very little about. Could it be that the risks of a homebirth that the medical profession raised concerns about were for the most part of their own doing? Is it possible that the hospital pathway of care, the lying in bed, breaking waters after an arbitrary time limit was met, for example, could actually be causing most of the problems that women now faced during childbirth?

In a bid to discover which is the safest place to give birth a massive study of nearly 65,000 women was carried out in England. Over a two year period the 'Birthplace in England' study looked at mother and baby complication rates for hospital consultant led units, hospital midwife led units, stand-alone birth centres and home births. Interestingly, the study found that women who had booked for a homebirth or into a midwifery led unit had a far lower experience of any medical intervention, for example Caesarean section, forceps or ventouse birth. The study further found that women having their first baby at home or in a midwifery led unit had a substantially higher rate of needing to be transferred into a consultant led unit than women who had given birth vaginally before. The majority of transfers were for pain relief or as a precaution measure because the baby had passed a bowel movement.

A consultant led unit proved the safest option for an expectant mother with complicated medical conditions, such as heart concerns or problems with their baby. Overall though, the research found that for women with a low risk in pregnancy and who had already had a vaginal birth, the safest place for mother and baby was a homebirth. Also, for women who were having their first baby and had been identified as having a low risk pregnancy, a midwifery led unit was equally safe as a consultant led unit to give birth for them and their babies.

Homebirth

The greatest benefits of a homebirth are the privacy and familiar environment. A midwife entering your home will tend to be more amenable to your wishes and less likely to leave you alone in labour, unless that is what you want. You will also be attended by two midwives when you enter active labour and certainly when giving birth. Exceptions to this rule would be in the case of a quick birth.

You should feel more in control and more confident in asking why certain things are being done. Your birth partner will probably feel a greater sense of control, which in turn allows them to support you more effectively.

You will have spent the majority of your early labour at home, re-organising areas and discovering the positions and the rooms in which you feel most comfortable. This time has allowed you to relax and produce the hormones to progress labour. Leaving this comforting environment can disrupt the fine balance of hormones and you may find that by the time you arrive at hospital your labour may have slowed.

How to Get a Homebirth - Knowing your Rights

Planning a homebirth when you have been classed as low risk is simple, just inform your community midwife that you've chosen a homebirth and they should organise the rest. As with many things in the NHS risk assessments need to be performed and this ensures both you and your baby's safety. A midwife will usually attend your home to ensure that there is enough space for their equipment and to plan for any possible transfers into hospital.

What you may not know however is that regardless of what information you receive from your midwife or obstetrician you have a legal right to give birth wherever you choose. It may be that your pregnancy and labour are high risk and your medical team are concerned that prompt medical help may not be immediately available, as it would be in a hospital. Because of this your midwife and obstetrician have a duty to inform you of all the risks that may occur at home and they may give this information bluntly to ensure that you understand these risks. Once they have given you this information and are happy that you do understand them, the decisions you make from there are informed decisions. If you are deemed to be high risk for labour and birth and opt for a home birth it is at this point that you will usually meet a Supervisor of Midwives who will discuss a birth plan with you and ensure that you were made aware of any risks at your meetings with your midwife and obstetrician.

Role of a Supervisor of Midwives

Every practising midwife in the United Kingdom has a named Supervisor of Midwives and they ensure the safety of mothers and their babies by monitoring a midwife's practice and ensuring that it is up to date. Each midwife will meet with their named supervisor once a year to discuss the previous year's practice and where they aim to be during the upcoming year. For midwives whose practice requires closer scrutiny the supervisor will work closely with them until they deem that they are competent to practice independently. Although most Supervisors of Midwives are employed by NHS hospitals, their role as a supervisor is out with the NHS.

In essence they have two hats and if you have concerns about any care you have received or have been told that you cannot have a homebirth then you can contact any supervisor of midwives at your hospital or the Local Supervising Authority (LSA).

Midwifery Led Units & Birth Centres

It may be that a homebirth is not right for you but you would prefer to avoid a clinical hospital environment. If this is the case you may wish to consider midwifery led units or birth centres.

These units have a homely feel to them. There is far less emphasis on medical procedures and intervention and because of this there is a minimum of medical equipment in the room. As the title suggests both the midwifery led units and birth centres have no doctors on the premises. They may be within a hospital and in close proximity to a consultant led unit or in the grounds of the hospital. Others may in fact be a considerable distance from the nearest hospital and because of this may have midwives with advanced skills that enable them to carry out ventouse births to avoid needing to transfer you to a hospital. It is mainly for this reason that these units are suitable only for women considered to be as low risk for birth.

Consultant Led Units

These units, like midwife led units and birth centres, are guidelines driven. There is a higher rate of intervention in these types of units because they deal in high risk births. In these units there is immediate access to life saving equipment and operating theatres, something that is not available in birth centres, midwife led units and at home.

Whatever your wish for your place of birth your midwife will be able to inform you fully of what is available in your area and also support you in your choices for the birth of your baby.

How to Feed Your Baby

If a medicine was invented that promised protection for newborns and their mothers against a host of diseases and illnesses, that was not only free but also perfectly balanced in nutrients, wouldn't people welcome it? Well, breast milk is just that.

This is not intended to promote breastfeeding at the expense of formula feeding, but to ensure that the decisions you make on the method of feeding your baby is informed. You should fully understand the benefits of breastfeeding before you decide against it. Undoubtedly there are downsides to breastfeeding, such as the mother being the only person able to do it. If, however, you look at this logically, nature has intended that mums provide this nourishment.

It is a time for rest, a time to bond with your infant and not be burdened by household chores. Let your partner do the housework whilst you care for the child.

I want you to imagine that it is two in the morning and you are awoken by baby's crying; you jump from your bed and race through to your kitchen to begin making up his feed. Throughout the time is takes to make it up he is crying continuously, your partner is doing their best to settle him but milk is all that will help. When you return to feed him he guzzles it down, you wind him, change his nappy and then both of you try to settle back to sleep.

Now imagine that you wake because you sense that your baby is also awake, you look to him and find that he is now rooting and is indeed awake. You lift him to you and begin to feed him, he finishes and you change his nappy and then settle back to sleep. During all of this your partner has not wakened because he has had no need to. You may find this sexist, but having only one of you having broken sleep makes sense, especially when you realise that the sleep you do get when breastfeeding is a deeper, more refreshing sleep; it has changed and is now in tune with your baby's.

The practicalities continue when you are out and about as you will not need a changing bag full of bottles, bibs, bottle warmers, formula, just a nappy, wipes and a nappy sack.

For all these benefits there are downsides, breastfeeding can be painful and may feel continuous. Breastfeeding in public can be off putting for some women and this limits where and when they go out. Your breasts can leak at the most inopportune times and breastfeeding bras are not de rigeur in the least. Then there is mastitis and engorgement and having to express milk even when you are away from baby to prevent the mastitis and engorgement. But with each of these ailments there are methods that can be used to alleviate the symptoms and if you are still undecided there are also these benefits too:

Breastfed babies may have better:

- Brain development.

Breastfeeding may also protect your baby against:

- Multiple sclerosis
- Acute appendicitis
- Tonsillectomy
- Obesity & Diabetes

Women who have breastfed are at lower risk of:

- Breast and Ovarian cancer
- Hip fractures and osteoporosis
- It may protect against Rheumatoid arthritis.

Apart from the fact that it is at the perfect temperature and free there is also the benefit that skin to skin contact has on bonding and colonising your baby's gut with bacteria. Another benefit is the extra calories that are used when breastfeeding and your womb contracting down more quickly following childbirth.

During a breastfeed the mother's antibodies are passed to her baby which not only protect him against infections but are also thought to kick start his immune system. Formula milk does not contain these antibodies and cannot be adapted to specific gestations of pregnancy. It is for that reason that…

Artificially fed babies are at greater risk of:

- Infections of the stomach and gut
- Chest infections

- Severe gut infections
- Bladder and kidney infections
- Ear infections
- Allergic diseases including eczema
- Diabetes
- Sudden infant death syndrome
- Childhood leukaemia.

Infant feeding is a very personal decision and once made should be respected. Never feel guilty or embarrassed about the method that you choose, it will after all be right for you as a mother and your family.

Packing your Bags

You will find many examples of what to take with you to hospital but what you may not find is exactly how to pack it. Your bag should be packed in the order that you need it, preferably with a separate bag for your baby's things. Ideally these should be packed and ready to go before thirty seven weeks of pregnancy.

Expect your stay in hospital to be anything from two to six hours following a straightforward birth to two to three days for a more complicated birth which may include a caesarean section. Bear in mind that there is limited room in most labour rooms and certainly on most postnatal wards. With this in mind pack only the essentials that you will need for a twenty four hour stay in hospital. Remember, you will have visitors and your partner who will be able to replenish your bag as required. Another thing to bear in mind is the size of the bags you take with you. Try to fit everything into as small a bag as possible and ask yourself if you absolutely require everything in it. For example, if your stay is less than twenty four hours it is highly unlikely that you will need breast pads until your milk supply comes in. If you do need to stay in longer, your partner can bring some in for you.

If you are being induced however, you may be in hospital for one or two days before your labour begins so you may need to pack more luxuries such as magazines, books and a few more clothes. Your bag should include the following and be packed in this order. The first item on the list should go at the bottom of your bag:

Your Bag

- Clothing to wear home
- 2 Button down night dresses
- Sanitary pads (1 pack)
- Flannel and toiletries
- An old towel
- 5 Pairs of large briefs
- Warm socks
- 2 Comfortable and supportive bras
- Plastic bag for soiled clothing
- Slippers and Dressing Gown
- Something comfortable for labour

Your Baby's Bag

- Cotton wool
- Blanket to wrap baby in*
- 3 Muslin cloths
- 6 Nappies
- 1 Hat (wool)
- 3 Vests (newborn size)
- 3 Sleepsuits (newborn size)

Your Small Bag

- Camera
- Magazines
- Medication
- Phone and charger
- Purse
- Sandwiches and drinks
- Aromatherapy oils
- Birth hypnosis C.D.
- Music
- Your hospital or maternity notes

*You may wish to sleep with this blanket before the birth to ensure you and your partner's scent is on it. This is particularly helpful if you and your baby are separated for any reason as it will help to establish bonding and attachment.

Tips for Dads and Partners

FROM POSITIVE PREGNANCY TEST TO 16 WEEKS

Before we even get to the labour part of your duties we need to go back to the beginning, you were after all fifty percent of the cause. Before your partner has even had a positive pregnancy test she may 'feel' pregnant and those 'feelings' are not altogether pleasant, for one she will feel exhausted. She will probably feel incredibly nauseous and may vomit periodically throughout the day. The nausea, vomiting and exhaustion usually lasts until twelve to sixteen weeks but the symptoms should not be underestimated, they can be debilitating. If you couple these symptoms with the fact that you will not have informed people of the pregnancy then you can see that she will not be receiving sympathy from anyone other than you.

So how can you help? Well at this stage it is really all about support and empathy. You may need to help more around the house and you should also encourage her to eat little and often. Eventually she will become accustomed to the perpetual nausea but until then she will need lots of support, love and attention.

16 WEEKS TO 26 WEEKS

From this point she should start to feel much better and her bump will be noticeable. She will also have so much more energy and be back to her usual self. Your twenty week anomaly ultrasound scan should be due in a few weeks and once that has confirmed that all is well with mum and baby you need to compile a shopping list. For all parents to be this has to be the most exciting part, when you realise that a baby is now tangible and you have less than twenty weeks to prepare.

Shopping for Baby

Please do bear in mind that most of the equipment and clothing that is listed on most websites and books are luxuries and on the whole unnecessary. You should avoid buying any clothes at all if you can as you will be inundated with them as gifts and usually in the 0-3 month age range. When it comes to buying vests and sleepsuits, unless he is estimated to be weighing more than five kilograms at birth then newborn size is sufficient. Equally, if he is estimated to be smaller than average you may wish to buy the following clothing in 'tiny baby' size. Expect him to outgrow his initial sleepsuits and vests in two to four weeks from his birth.

You will definitely need the following and most can be found perused, the NCT website is an excellent source of local sales:

THE PRAM

If you have a car it should fit easily into it. You may also find it useful to buy one that converts from a flat surface to a buggy and perhaps that incorporates a carry cot. It is not advised to leave him in a car seat for any longer than necessary as his spine needs to be as straight as possible. For that reason you should avoid prams that allow you to clip your car seat to a pram frame.

If you intend to walk a lot with him you may wish to consider a three wheeler as they are more manoeuvrable especially over uneven ground. Two handles rather than a single bar will also allow you to hang shopping bags from them and a basket underneath your pram is essential. One final point to consider is whether or not you plan to have another baby fairly quickly. If this is the case then you might consider prams that convert to a double buggy to avoid the need to buy another within a short period of time.

CAR SEAT

Do not buy a second hand car seat as you have no idea if it has been damaged in any way. A newborn baby should always travel in a rear facing car seat and preferably in the back seat. If he does need to travel in the front ensure that the air bag on the passenger side is switched off. Finally ensure that you read the instructions carefully in order that it is fitted properly.

THE COT

It is safest for your baby to sleep in your room for the first six months of his life but that does not mean that he has to sleep in a cot. He may be happier in a smaller cradle and being more compact will leave you with more room in your bedroom. If you buy a second hand cot you only need to ensure that you buy a new mattress and that it is thoroughly cleaned. You should avoid cot bumpers, pillows and duvets too as they may overheat your baby. Sleeping bags, ensuring that they are appropriate for your baby's weight are a godsend.

BABY INTERCOM

The current advice for caring for your baby is to have them close to you at all times, day and night. There are many benefits to this, especially with babies that struggle to settle on their own and for breastfeeding. If you decide not to you may need a method of ensuring that if your baby needs you that you can hear him. There are many types of baby intercoms that come in varying forms from the basic two way radio to colour monitors. If you live in a small flat they will probably be unnecessary.

BEDDING

- 4 Cellulose blankets
- 6 Sheets, fitted or flat
- Sleeping bags

CLOTHING

- 10 Newborn (up to four k.g.) vests or bodysuits,
- 10 Newborn sleepsuits
- 2 Woollen hats in winter
- 2 cotton hats in summer
- 2 cardigans
- 1 snow suit

OTHER EQUIPMENT

- Bottle Feeding:
- Steriliser and bottle brush
- 6 bottles
- Formula milk, powder and cartons

Breastfeeding:

- Breastpump
- Steriliser
- Stroller Blanket
- Baby blanket for you both to sleep with
- V-pillow or other breastfeeding pillow
- Baby Sling or carrier
- 20 Muslin cloths
- 10 Bibs
- 4 baby towels
- 4 flannels
- Top and tail bowl
- 4 large bags of cotton wool
- Room and bath thermometer
- Changing mat
- 2 packs of size 1 nappies

You do not need to buy these items but they may make your life simpler:

VIBRATING ROCKER

This will allow you to settle and soothe your baby without the need to constantly hold him. It will also allow you a greater degree of freedom as it can be moved easily throughout the home. You may also find these useful:

- Mobile
- Books
- Toys

You will probably never use these:
- Baby bath
- 0-3 month clothing

Things for Mum

This is certainly not the shopping trip of dreams but essential none the less. Your partner will definitely need the following but would probably prefer privacy when doing so. While she is doing this now might be a good time to do your own shopping and find that perfect present for her for after the birth of your baby.

- 2 packets of maternity pads
- 1 packet of breast pads, if breastfeeding
- 4 nursing bras
- 1 perineal gel ice pack (Boots or Mothercare)
- Large scarf to use during breastfeeding
- 4 Button down nightdresses
- 15 pairs of large briefs
- 1 Changing bag, preferably unisex
- Thank you cards and stamps

When you see this in list form it does look daunting and expensive but this equipment can be obtained at any time. Your pram, car seat and cot can be delivered at around thirty six weeks to prevent it cluttering your home while still allowing adequate time to familiarise yourself with them.

As the pregnancy progresses she will gradually feel more tired and uncomfortable. Nightly foot rubs and back massage are essential as is reassurance during this time.

36 WEEKS ONWARDS

The Checklist

Imagine for a moment that you have everything organised. The bags are all packed, the maternity notes are in a bag and the car seat is in the spare room. You're partner has decided that now is the time to leave for hospital. By this point panic may set in and invariably things not in plain sight may be forgotten.

The answer to this problem is a checklist. A printed copy is excellent but a handwritten list on an A4 sheet is just as effective and use as large a font as possible. The checklist will look something like this and should include everything you think you'll need for your time in hospital:

- Hospital bag
- Baby's hospital bag
- Your small bag
- Maternity notes
- Water and sandwiches from the freezer
- Phone and charger
- Laptop & Music
- House Keys
- Warm coat for birth partner

- Change for hospital parking
- Car seat in car

There are other things you may wish to add to this, for example, if you have a pet you may wish to add 'Feed Fish' to the list or if you are on medication add that to the list. When it is completed you should tape it to the inside of your front door, or back door if that is the one you intend to leave by. When you do eventually leave for the hospital you will take the list down and check through it just before you leave. This way you will have no concerns of forgetting important things like sandwiches.

On the subject of sandwiches, if you make up plain cheese or cold meat sandwiches they can be placed in the freezer in advance along with small bottles of water. Once removed from the freezer they will defrost in a short period of time and your food and water will always be chilled.

You also need to ensure that the following are done as these will be your sole responsibility:

- Ensure the car's fuel tank is full
- Put together the cot
- Put together the pram
- Service the car
- Familiarise yourself with the car seat
- Place car seat in the boot of the car
- Mattress pad on the back seat of your car
- Make up plain sandwiches and place in freezer
- Buy bottled water and place in freezer
- Compile your checklist
- Help to decorate the nursery

Chapter 6

Birth Plans

The importance of birth plans cannot be underestimated. They are an essential tool in making your midwife, and other healthcare providers aware of your preferences for labour and birth. That is not to say that they are set in stone, nor should they be. It is important to remember that it is not a list of what you 'want' to happen, merely a preference. However, the word 'plan' conveys an expectation that any birth can be planned and that is simply not true. We can plan for what we may need. To suggest that labour and its outcomes can be planned is setting women up for a negative birth experience and its accompanying anxiety.

A more appropriate name would be birth wishes and that is the way you should view your birth plan. They are a list of wishes, or preferences that your midwife is aware of and that she can advocate for on your behalf. The main pitfalls of birth plans are that they are heavily reliant on having a midwife complete one with you as you need to have their knowledge in order to complete one. If you don't have access to a midwife's time and specialist knowledge you become reliant on a birth plan template. You then have to complete it using predominantly inaccurate information from the internet, or worse, give up altogether.

This Book will help you make decisions about your birth plan but it is much more beneficial to have a midwife present at the time. There may be certain aspects of your pregnancy or labour that will require a bespoke birth plan service, especially if you are classed as 'high risk' due to a complicated pregnancy. To help with this, there is a 'birth wishes' template at the end of this chapter which should assist you in completing one. Put your name at the top of your birth plan and include the name you would prefer to be called. Once you are happy with the contents of it you should type it up, print it out on coloured paper and place it at the front of your notes ensuring that it is easily identified. Just remember in labour to point out your birth plan to your midwife and have it in the front of your notes if you can.

If you have set your mind on something, for example, having an epidural, it is important to convey that message to your midwife. In this instance it may be wise to write in your birth plan: 'I have read thoroughly on the subject of epidural and I am aware of their risks and benefits. I do not wish to be talked out of an epidural when I request one. I do however appreciate that the anaesthetist may be busy with an emergency at that point and accept that I may have to wait'. Midwives are constrained by guidance and statutory regulations. It would be remiss of them to provide you with pain relief without first ascertaining that you are aware of the procedure, its risks and benefits. By using this statement the midwife will be happy that you have made this decision with full understanding and at a time when you were able to think these decisions through clearly.

The next few pages concern your birth plan and how to complete it. It may be an idea at this point to have a pen handy to jot down your birth plan as you go on the handy 'birth plan notes' section.

How to Write a Birth Plan

Put your name at the top of your birth plan and include the name you would prefer to be called.

BIRTH PARTNER

Here you will put the name of your birth partner, their relationship to you and their contact details. This information helps your midwife to gauge the dynamics of the relationship more effectively and contact them for you if necessary.

BIRTH ENVIRONMENT

Here you will state what type of environment you would prefer. You should also state whether or not you wish assistance from your midwife to re-arrange the hospital room to accommodate these wishes.

MONITORING BABY'S HEARTBEAT

This is where you will explain your preferences for monitoring your baby's heartbeat. If you would prefer to have continuous monitoring then you would document this here. Please read the information on 'Monitoring Baby's heartbeat' before completing this though.

POSITIONS FOR LABOUR AND BIRTH

You should explain your preferences for an active or water birth here. You may also wish to add a request for your midwife to assist and encourage you to change positions and remain mobile. You may also wish to mention your preference for a position to give birth in. However, this usually becomes instinctive and you may find you use many different positions at this stage.

COPING WITH PAIN

Pain relief is a large subject and there is more information on this in the chapter 'helping to reduce anxiety and pain'. Here, you explain your preferences for pain relief in labour. You should try to use this as a way of informing your midwife of how you would like her to help you manage pain. Such as; 'I am aware of all methods of pain relief available to me and I would prefer my midwife not to mention or offer pain relief to me'. You should also try to avoid statement such as 'I do not, under any circumstances, want an epidural.' The reason for this is the impact this could have on you psychologically. If you have decided that an epidural is not for you, then simply put 'I do not plan on using an epidural for pain relief.' No one will force you into anything, especially if this is expressed in writing.

EPISIOTOMY AND TEARS

Here you will document your preferences for whether or not you would prefer to tear of have a surgical cut. Tears are extremely common with first babies and they do not hurt as they happen. As your baby's head is stretching your perineum you will feel a burning sensation and as your tear occurs that burning stops immediately. Tears can be placed into four categories depending on their severity; first degree, second degree, third degree and fourth degree.

A first degree tear involves just the skin of your perineum and if it is not bleeding you will not normally be advised to have it sutured. If you sustain a second degree tear the advice nowadays is that having it sutured reduces the risk of infection and allows it to heal quicker. If your tear is bleeding whether first or second degree you will be advised to have sutures as this will prevent you from having unnecessary blood loss. You will always have good pain relief while having your perineum repaired. Your legs will usually be placed in lithotomy poles, or stirrups and the repair itself usually takes around fifteen minutes and maybe sooner if the tear is small. The material that is used nowadays dissolves so there is no need to have the sutures removed.

Third and fourth degree tears involve the muscle that surrounds your back passage and in order to appose the muscle good lighting and pain relief are essential. Your obstetrician will want to take you to the operating theatre to carry this out.

Occasionally an episiotomy may be required. This is a surgical cut of your perineum to help you give birth. You will always be informed of why your midwife or obstetrician wishes to do it and they will obtain your consent before carrying out the procedure. They are no longer routine practice and local anaesthetic will always be used, although like tears they do not hurt as they happen.

There are only three reasons when an episiotomy may be required and these are;

- If you require a forceps birth, to provide adequate space.
- If your baby has become distressed and by doing one he will be born immediately.
- If you are giving birth to your baby in a breech position, again to allow space in your vagina.

If your midwife asks for your consent to perform one for any other reason, ask her why she feels it needs to be done because at present the current evidence and NICE guidelines do not support it in any circumstances other than those described above. It is also important to be aware that most evidence points to episiotomies actually increasing the risk or third degree tears.

There are however many techniques employed by midwives during your birth to minimise your chances of tearing but perineal massage is something that can be done at home by yourself.

Perineal Massage

Our risk of tearing is also predestined by genetics but there are some things that you can do to reduce that risk. These include; avoiding active pushing or 'Valsalva' manoeuvre' and pushing in any position other than on your back. There is also a growing body of evidence that supports the use of perineal massage as a way of reducing your risk of tearing. It is carried out antenatally from between thirty four to thirty six weeks.

You need to do this at least three times per week and for around three to five minutes at a time. First of all find some unscented oil such as massage oil and sit with your knees to the side or stand with a foot resting on a stool or chair. Using your thumbs, insert them into your vagina and then place your forefingers on the skin of your perineum. You now need to stretch this skin gently until you feel a burning sensation and repeat for around three to five minutes and do this at least three times per week. You should notice that the skin around your perineum has stretched over the course of a few weeks.

ASSISTED DELIVERIES AND CAESAREAN SECTION

The chapters covering assisted birth and caesarean section in emergencies will assist you to complete this. This topic allows you to document your preferences for the management of the procedures. You may wish to write that you wish your partner to accompany you to theatre. You should also avoid expressions such as 'I do not want', expand on this, such as writing 'I wish to avoid any intervention and would appreciate your help in achieving this'. Remember, your midwife or obstetrician will wish to avoid any unnecessary risks too.

SEX OF OUR BABY

This heading is for informing your midwife of whether or not you know the sex of your baby. State here who you would like to inform you of the sex when your baby is born.

SKIN TO SKIN CONTACT

Here you will document whether you wish skin to skin contact with your baby straightaway, or whether you wish your baby to be dried first.

There are numerous reasons why skin to skin contact immediately after your baby's birth should be the norm and not provided merely at your request. Midwives should be using this as their default method and not after a discussion on the subject. The only logical reasons why skin to skin contact wouldn't be carried out immediately are;

- At caesarean section where there are serious concerns about your baby and he needs to be assessed straightaway by paediatricians.
- If you have stipulated that you do not wish this.

All other methods of birth including forceps and ventouse should not prohibit skin to skin contact even if it is just for the time it takes to clamp and cut your baby's cord.

The reasons for this are that the benefits for such a simple thing are so great. Not only does skin to skin contact help with bonding and attachment in the early days and beyond it also helps to regulate your baby's breathing and temperature. Another benefit is that it allows your baby's skin to be colonised by your bacteria and this, plus breastfeeding are thought to be important in preventing problems with allergies and eczema later in life.

If you happen to have a baby who is in the neonatal unit or 'special care' then he will usually be cared for in an incubator as this allows mechanical control of his temperature. If he is premature this temperature is vitally important. However, by using skin to skin contact where possible you are still able to regulate his temperature and studies of baby's in the neonatal unit show that this kind of care or 'kangaroo care' can help to stabilise their oxygen levels too.

Skin to skin contact also benefits mothers who are breastfeeding. Babies who are left for at least one hour following their birth, in skin to skin contact, are more likely to latch on and feed without any assistance or problems. For those babies who have latched on with no problems, the added benefits are that breastfeeding is more easily established and women will have fewer problems with sore and cracked nipples.

CORD CLAMPING

Would you prefer to wait a few minutes to allow your baby to receive more of his blood from the placenta or would you prefer his cord to be clamped straightaway. If you wish your baby to have some of the benefits of a physiological third but wish to have active management you can opt for 'delayed cord clamping'. This involves placing your baby on your abdomen and then waiting one to three minutes before the cord is clamped and you are given drugs to contract your uterus. If you prefer to have your baby on your chest, because the blood flow has to work against gravity, it should be left slightly longer, up to five minutes before dividing the cord.

A review of research on this subject found that there was no significant difference between the groups having delayed and immediate cord clamping on the rate of severe blood loss. Furthermore, a Swedish randomised controlled trial in 2011 found that using delayed cord clamping reduced levels of babies with anaemia, or low iron count. It was also found to reduce the risk of babies suffering from iron deficiency at four months of age, a condition linked to poorer brain development.

Most concerns prior to this research centred around an increased iron level leading to higher levels of jaundice in babies. This study found that there was no significant increase in babies having polycythaemia, a high concentration of red blood cells in the blood. It also found no significant difference in babies with high levels of bilirubin in their blood, or jaundice that required treatment.

PLACENTA

This will explain whether or not you wish the injection to speed up the birth of your placenta or whether you would prefer to let it come away naturally.

Your placenta and membranes are around one third the weight of your baby but made entirely of soft tissue. The placenta itself is usually round in shape and anything from one to two centimetres thick. It has the 'maternal side' where it was embedded into the wall of your uterus and the 'foetal side' which contains the membranes, blood vessels and his umbilical cord. The side which embedded into your uterus did so within one week of conception and small blood vessels, called 'arterioles' spread out from your blood supply to feed this newly forming placenta.

Newborn babies have a tiny amount of blood in their bodies, the average amount being seventy to eighty five millilitres per kilogram. Therefore a baby weighing three kilograms will have just over two hundred and fifty millilitres or half a pint. If the baby's cord is clamped and cut straightaway, up to one third or eighty millilitres can be left in the placenta. Added to that, the remainder in the placenta, which will be simply thrown away with other 'clinical waste', will also include iron stores and stem cells. Like adults, newborns will be affected by any loss of blood.

If you lose blood giving birth it may make you feel tired, weak and your pulse may rise and your blood pressure drop. The drop in blood pressure is a direct result of your body suddenly being deprived of fluid, or blood, and that loss of fluid equals a loss of pressure in your blood vessels. This however does not explain fully the rise in your pulse and the feeling of weakness and tiredness. These are a direct consequence of losing the haemoglobin molecules in your blood. Haemoglobin is the oxygen transport blood vessel and the less of this you have in your blood the quicker your heart has to pump to deliver the remaining oxygen filled haemoglobin to your muscles and other cells. Your body recognises that it already has to work harder to transport less oxygen and it forces you to rest. That is the reason your heart rate, or pulse will rise and you feel weak and tired.

If you are of an average size then during pregnancy the amount of blood in your body will have increased from around four and a half litres to six litres. This happens to ensure that your body functions normally as it diverts extra blood to your uterus.

Physiological 3rd Stage of Labour

This method is the most natural way of delivering your placenta and involves placing your baby on your abdomen or chest for skin to skin contact and waiting for your placenta to be expelled. Once your baby is born a chain reaction takes place in his and your bodies which causes the placenta to peel away from the wall of your uterus.

Oxytocin is the main protagonist of this reaction and for this reason it is wise to latch your baby to your breast for his first feed. Skin to skin contact will also help and if you are not planning to breastfeed then simply rolling your nipples will also have the desired effect. As this happens you will notice that the cord becomes pale and has stopped delivering blood to your baby. Around the same time your midwife will notice a loss of blood from your vagina. The blood loss is from you, from the wound on the wall of your uterus as the arterioles and their blood supply are slowly cut off. Your uterus and nature are amazing. A few seconds earlier half a litre of blood per minute was flowing to your placenta. Once your placenta has come away from your uterus, the muscles, into which these arterioles burrowed, begin to contract again. This contraction of the uterine muscle constricts the blood vessels between the muscle fibres, known as 'living ligatures', and stops the bleeding.

As your uterus begins to contract you will feel what are known as 'after pains' in your lower abdomen and will start to feel a heaviness in your bottom. This heaviness is your placenta as it is forced out of your uterus and into your vagina in much the same way as your baby was. When you feel this pressure your midwife will ask you to push down and your placenta will just come away. The whole process usually takes between fifteen and twenty minutes.

When undertaking physiological management it is important that your midwife does not use a mixture of the two approaches as this has been shown to cause an unnecessarily heavy blood loss. With physiological management of the third stage the cord, where possible, should not be touched until your placenta has delivered. If you have not passed your placenta within one hour it would be sensible to empty your bladder if you have not already done so. This and the action of your baby breastfeeding will usually cause your body to expel it.

There are occasions where hospital guidelines advocate the use of active management in pregnancy which has a high risk of blood loss. These would include twin pregnancy and pregnancies affected by polyhydramnios (above normal levels of fluid surrounding baby) or any other where the uterus has been overly distended.

Active 3rd Stage of Labour

The other method of delivering your placenta is known as 'active management'. This involves giving an injection of syntocinon or syntometrine into a muscle after your baby is born. This is used 'prophylactically' as there will not yet have been any bleeding. It can also be used to treat some causes of bleeding following a physiological third stage or heavy bleeding following active management. Syntocinon is a synthetic form of oxytocin and syntometrine has another component, ergometrine maleate added to it. Syntometrine can cause vomiting and raised blood pressure and has a higher rate of retained placenta, where there is difficulty removing the placenta. The difference between the two drugs in terms of blood loss over twenty four hours is negligible. Considering the side effects and risk factors of using syntometrine, many midwives and obstetricians have moved away from it and no longer use it routinely. If you already have high blood pressure, a heart problem or you wish to avoid the risk of vomiting you will only be offered syntocinon.

After waiting for signs that your placenta has separated your midwife will place one hand on your lower abdomen and with the other, pull the umbilical cord and deliver your placenta. With this method the whole process is usually complete within five to ten minutes and blood loss at that time is shown in studies to be less than with a physiological third stage. However, clamping of the umbilical cord is done before your baby's cord has stopped pulsating

A recent review of different studies comparing active and physiological management found that all women in these studies that underwent active management had less severe bleeding and low iron levels. However this was tempered by an increase in their blood pressure, more after pains, nausea and vomiting and an increase in the need for pain relief afterwards. It was also noted that with this group that there was a higher rate of re-admission to hospital with vaginal bleeding and a reduction in the birth weight of their babies.

The increase in re-admission to hospital with bleeding was thought to be related to the body's ability to regulate the amount of blood that it now needs in a non-pregnant state. By limiting the blood loss at birth using drugs merely increased the risk of heavier blood loss later at home. The reduction in the birth weight of babies was also thought to be a result of the loss of up to eighty millilitres of blood left in the placenta due to early clamping and cutting of his cord.

When the researchers then looked at only those women categorised as low risk, who lost up to one litre of blood after delivering their placenta, they found no significant difference between both the active and physiological management groups. Research has also shown that in the developed world women can cope with blood loss of up to one litre without coming to serious harm.

FEEDING OUR BABY

Here you will document how you plan to feed your baby and whether or not you would like assistance with this.

VITAMIN K

You should document here whether or not you wish your baby to have Vitamin K and how you wish it administered.

The Department of Health recommend that all babies are given a vitamin K supplement at birth and this comes in two forms: A one off injection into your baby's muscle or a course of oral medication given at birth and then subsequent doses up to one month depending on which method of feeding you are using.

We all need vitamin K to help our blood clot and most of this is taken in by our diet or produced in our gut by bacteria. As babies are yet to establish feeding, their guts are totally sterile and will have no bacteria so are born with very low levels of vitamin K in their bodies.

On very rare occasions, one in ten thousand babies will be born with insufficient vitamin K in their bodies to control even the smallest of bleeds. This is known as vitamin K deficiency bleeding and can cause babies to bleed from their mouth, nose and even into their brain where it may cause brain damage and in extremely rarely death. It usually occurs from around three to six days of age but may also happen later. This risk can be reduced to one in a million babies simply by giving a vitamin K supplement.

The decision surrounding whether you want your baby to have this supplement or not and by which route will be yours, providing he is well. It may be that you dislike the thought of an injection but your baby's stomach does not absorb the vitamin K supplement very effectively. Because of this he is at slightly greater risk of developing vitamin K deficiency bleeding with the oral supplement.

FOLLOWING THE BIRTH

This is where you may wish to express your preference for having some private time as a family and how quickly following the birth you wish to go home.

Your Birth Plan Template Notes

BIRTH PARTNER

BIRTH ENVIRONMENT

MONITORING BABY'S HEARTBEAT

POSITIONS FOR LABOUR AND BIRTH

COPING WITH PAIN

EPISIOTOMY AND TEARS

SEX OF OUR BABY

SKIN TO SKIN CONTACT

CORD CLAMPING

PLACENTA

FEEDING OUR BABY

VITAMIN K

FOLLOWING THE BIRTH

Chapter 7

Problems with your Pregnancy

As much as we all wish for a straightforward pregnancy, labour and birth there are occasions where this just may not be the case. That is not to say that these problems are insurmountable just that they will require you to deal with your pregnancy and labour in a different way. Some of these problems may be identified early on in your pregnancy as you may have been screened for them. Others will become apparent because they will either make you feel unwell or the problem will be apparent to you in other ways. If you have had a problem identified in your pregnancy then you will already be receiving specialist care.

If you notice any of the following problems please contact your midwife or hospital straightaway. If a problem is noticed in the middle of the night your maternity notes should tell you who to call. If you are in any doubt as to who this may be the safest thing to do is to contact your labour ward.

Baby's Moving Less

There are many reasons why baby's movements may change or slow down during the day. The most obvious one is, like the rest of us, that they need a sleep. Another reason is that they may change from kicks to stretches usually due to the baby having less room. As your pregnancy progresses and especially after 26 weeks you should notice that there is a pattern to your baby's movements. They may be extremely active when you wake up, less active at lunchtime and again extremely active in the afternoon and evening.

Midwives and obstetricians used to advise women to count their baby's kicks and ten a day was the minimum. The problem with that method was that for the very active baby's their movements had actually reduced. For some women that would lull them into a false sense of security. There was also confusion surrounding whether it was ten kicks or ten patterns of movements. Babies, when they become distressed will conserve all their energy and they do not need contractions to become distressed. For some babies the placenta just does not work efficiently enough or there may be other problems that need to be addressed.

A baby that is healthy and not distressed will keep to that same pattern of movements. Providing the pattern is consistent there is no need to listen to your baby's heart beat at your antenatal appointments. However, some women do wish to have this and can request that their midwife listens to his heart beat for them.

A Note of Caution.

If your baby's movements have slowed down please don't be tempted to listen to your baby's heart beat yourself for reassurance. Even the most distressed baby's will have a heartbeat and it will fluctuate greatly as they try to compensate for the problem. The longer you leave this the greater the chance of ignoring a serious problem. If you notice that your baby is moving less frequently than normal then please contact either your midwife or your labour ward straightaway.

Bleeding From Your Vagina

This is not to be confused with your 'show' which is the mucus plug of your cervix. When your 'show' comes away it is usually a dark red or brown and mixed with mucous. When you bleed from your vagina it is fresh, red blood which varies in the amount. It is a warning sign and you should inform your labour ward or midwife straightaway. Again there are many reasons why this would occur and it may happen with or without pain. The most common reason for bleeding is that there is an area of raw skin on your cervix which bleeds easily, especially after intercourse although not always. Another reason may be that your placenta is low lying and very close to or covering your cervix and may cause heavier blood loss. If this has been identified earlier in pregnancy you will have been made aware of this eventuality and what to do.

A much rarer reason for bleeding is where the placenta has begun to come away from the wall of the uterus. It happens in one half to two percent of pregnancies. It is usually accompanied by constant abdominal pain and then tightening of your uterus or contractions. You may also feel that your uterus is tense most of the time. The amount of blood loss can vary and in some instances there is none, which is known as concealed. If you experience any of these symptoms you should contact your labour ward straightaway. If the bleeding is running down your legs then you need to phone an ambulance immediately.

Many people think that a baby's and mother's blood circulate together and that they are mixed. They are actually two separate circulations and the exchange of oxygen, waste and nutrients takes place at the placenta. Essentially the mother takes in oxygen and energy for her baby and removes all of her baby's waste products with her own; the one exception is if there has been some sort of trauma or bleed.

Rhesus negative mothers

If you are a rhesus negative blood group any bleeding in pregnancy and labour could potentially cause your baby's blood to mix with yours. If you are rhesus negative then molecules in your blood do not have a protein coat like those of people having a rhesus positive blood group.

If your baby is rhesus positive then their molecules would have a protein coat. Problems occur when the mother's immune system identifies one of the baby's blood molecules as a foreign body. Her body will then produce antibodies and these antibodies may attack a potentially healthy baby in a future pregnancy. Having an anti D immunoglobulin, or Anti D injection shortly after any bleeding protects against this. It is important to remind your midwife or obstetrician after any episode of bleeding or after giving birth that you are rhesus negative. It is always important to know your blood group.

Waters Breaking Before Labour

Your waters are made up of two membranes that sit together. The amnion is the thinner of the two membranes and is next to your baby and the thicker chorion membrane sits against your uterus. These membranes protect your baby and contain the fluid around him. They are not impermeable and microscopic organisms or germs can pass through them and enter the fluid, potentially causing an infection. Your body combats this by increasing the amount of discharge your vagina produces and altering its environment to limit the transit of these germs. Introducing anything into your vagina, such as fingers or a speculum instrument if the waters have broken, increases the risk of introducing infection.

Your membranes or waters have to break at some point in labour to allow your baby to be born. A 'forewater rupture' is when the membranes break in front of baby's head at the cervix. When the membranes break elsewhere is it called a 'forewater rupture'. You will experience a 'gush' with a forewater rupture and a trickle in the case of a hindwater.

This in and of itself is not a problem as long as the waters that come away are light pink or clear. If they are brown, green or yellow then it usually signifies that your baby has opened his bowels and passed meconium. Most babies with a mature gut and past their due date will pass meconium. It is no longer thought to be an indication that a baby is distressed. However midwives and obstetricians want to avoid your baby inhaling meconium and they are at risk of doing so if they are very distressed. The only way to reassure everyone that your baby is healthy, happy and only having a normal level of labour stress is to perform a trace of your baby's heart rate known as a cardiotocograph or heart rate trace. This will be explained in greater detail in the Chapter *'What to Expect in Hospital'*.

If the heart rate trace is normal then the meconium is of little concern. This surveillance can only be carried out in hospital so you should contact your labour ward or midwife if you experience coloured fluid.

Fluid stained with blood also needs to be checked out in hospital for the same reason as the 'bleeding from your vagina' section. If you experience blood stained fluid you should contact your midwife or labour ward straightaway.

The National Institute of Clinical Excellence (NICE) is an independent organisation set up by the Government in 1999. Its role is to analyse the research on drugs and treatments and to devise guidelines for their use within the NHS. NICE recommends that labour should be induced if it has not commenced 24 hours after waters have broken. Induction of labour is advised after this period because without the protective membranes the risk of infection increases.

Research shows the risk of your baby developing an infection that will require treatment when the waters break is approximately half of one percent, or one in two hundred babies. This risk increases to one percent or one in one hundred babies by twenty four hours. Although the risk doubles it remains a statistically small figure.

You will be asked to decide whether you want to have your labour artificially accelerated. This is done using a hormone drip, known as syntocinon and can be started straightaway or delayed for 24 hours to see if your labour starts on its own. If you do decide to have the hormone drip option then there is an increased risk that you may need an assisted birth. There is, however, no increase in the risk of needing a Caesarean section whether you delay this or not.

You also need to be aware that around 60 percent of women's labour will start naturally within 48 hours of their waters breaking. Therefore by waiting twenty four hours you may avoid the intervention of the hormone drip infusion. Information on the hormone drip can be found in the Chapter, *'Having your Labour Induced'*.

Whilst waiting for labour to begin naturally you should inform your midwife or labour ward if the following happen:

- Your baby's movements reduce.
- Your waters change colour.
- Your waters begin to smell.
- You feel unwell, hot or feverish.

Personal hygiene is also important to prevent infection and the following is advised:

- Change your sanitary towels frequently, at least every four hours.
- Do not use tampons
- Avoid bath foam or oils if you take a bath
- Avoid swimming.
- Refrain from sex until after your baby is born.

There are risks and benefits to both being induced immediately after your waters break and waiting for your labour to start naturally and you shouldn't be swayed either way. Do bear in mind, however, that occasionally the labour ward may be busy. During these times they may avoid inducing and accelerating women's labour to ensure that women in active labour are not redirected to another hospital.

If your membranes have been ruptured for over 24 hours before the birth of your baby the midwife may wish to monitor him for signs of infection after he is born. The length of time this monitoring takes varies between hospitals but the average is 24 to 36 hours.

During that period his temperature, heart rate, breathing rate and general wellbeing will be observed regularly on the postnatal ward. If there is anything suggestive of a possible infection then he will be assessed by the paediatricians who may advise antibiotics.

If you request an accelerated labour and it has not been immediately possible, and you have concerns regarding this, you should inform the midwife in charge of labour ward. Alternatively you could request to speak to the most senior obstetrician available.

Feeling Unwell

We all feel unwell at some point in our life and pregnancy is no different. In fact, women's immune systems are suppressed in pregnancy and they are more likely to catch infections and suffer more severe symptoms. For this reason women are advised to be vaccinated against influenza during the flu season.

Likewise, there are seasonal infections such as gastroenteritis and colds amongst others.

Symptoms of gastroenteritis include stomach cramps, nausea, vomiting and diarrhoea. It is dehydration caused by these that gives cause for concern. Therefore, you should contact your midwife or labour ward for advice if you feel unwell during your pregnancy.

Abdominal Pain

In the majority of cases abdominal pain is nothing more than the normal adjustments the body makes in pregnancy but any abdominal pain should be treated with caution. It is for that reason that you are advised to contact your midwife or labour ward for reassurance or treatment.

Rashes and Itching

Rashes and itching are another common ailment in pregnancy and are usually relatively minor. Normally they are relieved by wearing loose, natural clothing, cool baths and topical lotions such as calamine.

One notable exception to this is Obstetric Cholestasis which is a build-up of bile salts in your body. The symptoms of this are severe generalised itching, usually without a rash. It is wisest to discuss any itching with your midwife and she should be able to advise you as to whether you need to have tests to rule out Obstetric Cholestasis or treatment and advice for another ailment.

Chest Pain

Any chest pain at any point in your life should be taken seriously. You may find that the pain makes breathing in difficult or you may feel a constant pain. There is no way for your midwife or obstetrician to make an assessment and diagnosis without seeing you. In order to rule out extremely rare complications they will ask that you attend hospital to be assessed.

Difficulty Breathing

Also referred to as 'shortness of breath' and you may see it abbreviated to SOB. Like chest pain there can by many causes for this and your midwife or obstetrician will be unable to make an assessment or diagnosis without seeing you. If you do suffer from chest pain or shortness of breath in pregnancy it is important to inform your midwife or labour ward straightaway.

Dizziness, Double Vision, Swelling & Headaches

The drop in blood pressure in pregnancy makes most women feel faint in the early stages. However, later on in pregnancy episodes of fainting are fairly rare.

Dizziness, especially in the second half of your pregnancy can have numerous causes. It may be due to raised blood pressure. If your blood pressure is higher than your body is used to then it can lead to headaches and dizziness. You may also notice swollen hands and feet, especially towards the end of pregnancy.

In rare cases symptoms of swollen hands and feet may be caused by pre-eclampsia. This condition is not fully understood but is thought due to the constriction of uterine blood vessels, which feed the placenta. For some reason these, along with other blood vessels, narrow which means pressure has to increase to force the blood through these restricted vessels. The resulting increase in blood pressure causes headaches, dizziness, swelling all over the body and occasionally pain under the ribs. You will usually also begin to pass protein in your urine.

There are degrees of pre-eclampsia, ranging from mild to severe. In its mildest form your blood pressure and urine would be checked regularly along with certain blood tests.

Very rarely women can suffer from severe pre-eclampsia which effects up to one to two percent of pregnancies. If you suffer from this you would be admitted to hospital. Pre-eclampsia is relatively easy to diagnose and it is important that you inform your midwife or labour ward if you begin to suffer from any of these symptoms. If you begin to suffer from all of these symptoms the quicker you can have the condition diagnosed and treated the better.

Labour Before 37 Weeks of Pregnancy

Babies born before 37 weeks' gestation are classed as premature or pre term. Added concern is that all of their organs, to varying degrees, are immature and the earlier they are born the more potential problems they may have. Labour for any baby is stressful but the process prepares your baby's body to breathe for itself. Up until birth your baby's lungs have never been inflated and are full of fluid. The stress of labour causes the baby to absorb this fluid and kick starts the production of pulmonary surfactants, which help to keep the gas absorbing parts of the lungs open.

With this in mind any labour that begins before 37 weeks gestation should always be closely monitored. In most cases obstetricians and paediatricians may wish to give you steroids to help to mature your baby's lungs.

You may also be started on a drip in an attempt to slow down or halt labour long enough to allow the steroids time to work. Therefore, the sooner you can get to hospital the quicker the medical team there can identify what treatment you require. If your baby is born before 37 weeks you may have to stay in hospital longer than you anticipated.

If you have a very premature baby then he will be admitted to the neonatal unit or special care baby unit. As cots on these units offer very specialised care they are at a premium. It is important to bear in mind that if you attend in threatened or premature labour that you may be transferred to a more specialised unit. This will depend on your stage of labour and whether your hospital has the facilities to care for a baby of that gestation.

In these rarest of instances all efforts are made to transfer you to as close a unit as possible, but depending on the level of care required you may have to travel further than you would like. The simplest way to deal with this situation once you are in hospital is to focus on the main goal which is the best care for your baby. As soon as it is possible your baby will be transferred back to the nearest hospital from home.

Summary

You should contact your labour ward or midwife straightaway in the following circumstances:

- Your pattern of your baby's movements have stopped, reduced or slowed down
- You have a small amount of bleeding from your vagina
- Your waters have broken
- You feel unwell
- You have itching
- You have abdominal pain
- You have a headache, dizziness, swelling or double vision
- You have any type of vaginal discharge other than creamy or white.
- If you think you may be in labour before 37 weeks gestation
- If you have difficulty breathing

You should call a 999 ambulance if you experience any of the following:

- Bleeding from your vagina that is running down your legs
- Severe abdominal pain
- You have all four symptoms of pre-eclampsia – dizziness or headache and swelling and double vision and abdominal pain.
- Severe difficulty breathing
- Chest pain

Chapter 8

Support in Pregnancy, Labour & Birth

Role of the Birth Partner

Birth partners are exactly what they sound like, a partner in your birth. They can be anyone who can support and encourage you, empathise with you and who you trust to have your best interests at heart. You should put a great deal of thought into who you would like as your birth partner and whether or not you would like to have more than one. You may wish for your husband, boyfriend, or partner, to be present for the birth of your baby but worry that he will find it difficult to watch you in labour. In view of that you may decide that you would like a friend that has recently given birth to support you along with your partner.

The benefits of having someone who has recently given birth or who has previously supported someone else giving birth is that they know what to expect and are able to reassure you. They are also able to reassure your partner that certain aspects of labour are perfectly normal.

However, you need to avoid what is known as the 'nosey partner'. This is someone who has never witnessed a birth and wishes to experience someone give birth. Although they may be well-meaning they tend to be overcome by the rollercoaster of emotions in labour. Because of this they can occasionally neglect their primary role as birth support and may be unable to give you the reassurance that someone who has already witnessed or experienced a birth can.

Another pitfall is using someone who has had a particularly traumatic birth. They may begin to focus on the negative aspects of their birth and push alternatives as a way of helping you avoid a similar experience. They may also have their judgement clouded about certain aspects of care which may be inappropriate for your labour. A birth partner also needs to be aware of the length of time that they may be required to stay awake. Pregnant women have spent months becoming accustomed to varying degrees of sleep deprivation and a few more days of this in labour does little to faze them.

Birth partners on the other hand, especially those who have never witnessed a labour or birth may be wholly unprepared for this. Having two birth partners allows them to take sleep breaks and ensure that the other is cared for. As you will be focussing on your own labour it is important that your birth partner recognises and ensures that you are fed and kept hydrated. It is also vital that they make sure that they eat and drink and have regular breaks themselves.

During labour you do not have the emotional energy to worry about your partner and how they are coping.......so don't, they're there to support you!

Make sure that your second birth partner (the one who has experienced labour) is aware of what you want. Discuss your birth plan with them beforehand and give them clear roles, such as asking them to also take care of your partner and listen to their concerns too.

You may also wish them to advocate on you and your partner's behalf which will take some of the pressure from your partner. Do bear in mind however that legally the only person who can give consent for treatment is you. Staff will discuss things with you both but ultimately it must be you that gives consent. If, for any reason you are incapacitated then the medical staff will do whatever is in your best interests. This will all be discussed with your partner but they will not be asked to give consent on your behalf, which prevents the consequences of that decision affecting you both.

If you feel confident that your partner is able to cope with the role of birth partner then the privacy of you as a couple experiencing this journey is far more fulfilling. If on the other hand you feel that your partner may need to share the load and you cannot think of an appropriate second birth partner you may wish to consider the services of a doula.

Doulas provide a supportive, informative and nurturing role in childbirth and will advocate on your behalf. They have training in the birth process and are used to working closely with midwives and the rest of the labour ward team. They would also offer you support at home too in the early stages of labour.

Whether you decide to have a friend, relative, partner or doula in a supporting role it is important that they are aware of their role and what is expected:

- They should have read and understood your birth plan.

- They must ensure that the birth environment is as perfect as possible.
- They should ensure that you have enough to eat.
- Encourage you to drink often and to try to empty your bladder at least every four hours
- Encourage you to change positions to the one where your contractions are most effective.
- Provide back pain relief by rubbing your back or ensuring that the wheat bag or hot water bottle are warm.
- Encourage you to use all methods of non-medical pain relief available prior to stronger methods.
- Discourage you from lying or sitting down, especially if it reduces the frequency of the contractions.
- Use a calm, soothing and quiet voice and limit any unnecessary conversation.
- Offer physical support, if needed.
- Encourage you to keep going no matter how tired you become.
- If they are having difficulty watching you in pain they should keep it to themselves and do not raise the issue with you.
- If things are not going to plan explain this to you clearly and tell you what is recommended but avoid the temptation to make the decision for you.
- Make sure they have regular breaks.

When labour begins it normally builds up gradually and this gives your partner a chance to acclimatise to their role as a birth partner. Even if they are not to be the primary birth partner at these early stages, if they wish to, they can take on that role until you feel ready to call for your other birth partner. In order to prepare them for this ask them to read the following pages, it will enlighten them.

For Your Partner

You will have completed all your tasks and you are now waiting patiently for labour to begin. When it does happen keep calm and keep smiling. There are many things about your partner's imminent behaviour that may shock and surprise you and it is important that you do not convey that to her in any way.

You are not expected to empathise with the pain of every contraction and nor should you. If your partner feels that she can cope on her own for a while then don't feel guilty, go to bed and get some rest. Women have been prepared for the sleep deprivation involved in labour, men have not. Encourage her to drink throughout labour and offer her food and remember to do so yourself. When your partner's contractions become intense she will need you to be strong, supportive and reassuring. With that in mind under NO circumstances do the following:

Avoid

- Do not tell your partner (or your midwife) that 'she is tired'

- Equally heinous is telling your partner (or your midwife) that she is 'in too much pain' or 'cannot do this any longer.
- And never, ever tell anyone how tired or how much pain you are in – you will be summarily tortured by all.

On a serious note, labour is mentally similar to running a marathon. All positive aspects must be reinforced and there is no place for negative thoughts. Most importantly, when you are watching your partner in pain ask yourself this question. '*Is this upsetting my partner, can she no longer cope or is it me that it is upsetting and can I no longer cope?*' If it is the latter, remember that your partner does not have the emotional time to worry about how you are coping. Have a hard word with yourself and tell yourself to get a grip. Then, tell your partner how strong and amazing she is, because she is, and she is doing all this for you and your baby.

Once you are on a labour ward the atmosphere may change and you may find it more challenging to question situations that you are unsure or unhappy about. You are your partner's advocate so make sure that your midwife understands your partner's birth plan and any wishes for the birth. There may be occasions when your midwife or obstetrician discusses with you both possible interventions that may be needed, for example the hormone drip. This may make you feel overwhelmed with responsibility. In order to ensure that you both have all the information needed to make informed choices use the following mnemonic device to ask the following questions of the proposed treatment:

B.R.A.I.N.

B **Benefits** of the proposed treatment or intervention?

R **Reasons** it may be needed?

A **Alternatives** to the proposed interventions?

I **Instincts**, what does your partner feel she wants to do?

N **Nothing**, if you don't act what will happen?

By using this questioning tool you will be able to ascertain whether or not the intervention is entirely necessary and be reassured as to the reasons for it. During this discussion ensure that your partner has heard and understands the information and ask her to make the final decision.

PART 2

Giving Birth

Chapter 9

Early Labour at Home

As with any labour, providing everything is progressing normally with your pregnancy and no complications have been identified then you should aim to stay at home for as long as possible. The only exception to that would be where women have had complications identified in their pregnancy. Those women should contact their local maternity unit for specific advice when they think that their labour has started. You may also feel that the day you give birth will never arrive and this can be aggravated by the due date.

The Myth of the Due Date

At your first appointment or ultrasound scan your midwife or obstetrician will have given you a due date or an estimated date of delivery. You may occasionally hear this referred to as E.D.D. but the number of women who actually give birth on that date is only about two in every hundred so it's really not that accurate.

A due date is useful as it simplifies the organisation and planning of your care. After all, it is much easier for your midwife and obstetrician to calculate a set amount of time from a given date. For you though this date looms with excitement and anticipation in equal measure, but when it passes you feel deflated and disappointed. For other women the two week wait following their due date can prove so frustrating and mentally arduous that they begin to question their body's ability to function effectively.

It would be more sensible to provide you with a 'labour window', a point in time when you are most likely to labour spontaneously. That window would be from thirty seven weeks gestation until forty two weeks gestation. Anything earlier and your baby would be classed as premature and later post mature. With this information you can plan your life more effectively and you can avoid fixating on one arbitrary point in time. When your labour finally begins it will feel neither unexpected nor elusive.

Alternatively you could add two weeks to your estimated due date and call it your 'best before' date and also tell friends and family that date. Not only will this help you avoid the negative thoughts of going past your due date but also limit annoying texts and phone calls as your due date approaches.

What are Contractions?

When labour does finally begin your first clue will be period type cramps that will come in waves and coincide with your uterus tightening. Essentially these are Braxton Hicks, but the sensation may now be accompanied by pain which may also be felt in your back. They will be irregular to start with, coming every twenty minutes, then every four minutes and back up to six, and probably last for 20-30 seconds at a time. In the meantime your cervix is softening and shortening from around 3cm long to paper thin and you will feel the pain centrally in your lower abdomen.

Over time, and it may be a few days of stopping and starting, you will find they begin to arrive like clockwork; this is what is meant by the term 'regular'. Their intensity increases and the sensation becomes more noticeable over your entire uterus and they last for more than 60 seconds. You need not time all the contractions but when you contact your midwife or labour ward you will be asked about their frequency. It is good to have an idea of this as it will help them assess whether you can stay at home longer.

There are no hard and fast rules regarding the frequency of contractions but suffice to say that once they are regular you should be having approximately three every ten minutes, lasting for over a minute. They may be more or less frequent than this. You should no longer be able to talk through them and you will be struggling to cope at the height of the contraction. You are the best judge of how long you wish to stay at home. Research has shown that if you are classed as low risk you undergo less intervention the less time you spend in hospital. You will also find that you are more likely to have a shorter, less painful labour at home because of the comfortable environment.

How to Know When You Are in Labour

There are three stages of labour, First, Second and Third. These stages are further split into sub-stages.

First Stage – Latent Phase

This phase of labour has the slowest build up and starts with your first contraction. You would normally be assessed to be in the latent phase of labour if your cervix is yet to thin out completely, your contractions are yet to become regular and your cervix is not opening or dilating, or doing so slowly. As this stage can take longer the active phase of labour it can be an incredibly frustrating time and best served in the comfortable surroundings of home.

Signs of Active Labour

There is no definitive way to ascertain whether or not you are in active labour. Labour in general is much simpler to quantify. If you are having painful contractions then you are, by definition, in labour. As a general rule you will normally be advised to contact your midwife or labour ward if you experience the following:

- Painful contractions.
- Contractions coming every three minutes or more.
- Contractions that have become regular.
- Contractions now lasting at least sixty seconds.
- Unable to talk through your contractions at the height of them.
- Need for stronger pain relief.
- Pressure in your back passage similar to needing to open your bowels.
- An overwhelming urge to push.

- Wanting to push to get comfortable.
- A heavier bloody 'show'.

Every woman is different and even with all of these signs it may well be that labour cannot be established. Equally, it may be that you are one of the few women who will experience no pain in labour. You should still have contractions. Do not be too concerned with this, but if you are in any doubt telephone your midwife or labour ward for advice.

First Stage – Active Phase

- Your contractions have become regular.
- You are no longer able to talk through them.
- They will last for around one minute.
- You may begin to feel pressure in your bottom similar to the sensation when you need to open your bowels.
- The pain with your contractions is now all over your uterus.
- You become more focused and withdrawn.

As you move into the active phase of your labour you will notice that your contractions become gradually more frequent, more intense and last longer. It is at this point that most women will start to waiver and fear they cannot cope with the intensity of labour. After all, labour is not without pain, it is a very powerful experience but it is rarely, ever more than you can bear. You may feel that if the next contraction is stronger or longer then you will not cope, but that point will usually never come.

What you have to remember is that as your body is producing these huge quantities of oxytocin it is also producing vast quantities of endorphins, your natural pain killer. The more oxytocin you produce the more endorphins you produce, therefore as your labour becomes more intense your body produces more endorphins. This is why you never have to fear the next contraction or organise pain relief in advance *'just in case'*. If you have managed through the contractions in the latent phase of labour with minimal pain relief it will be no different in the active phase.

At this point, and throughout, your birth partners will be reinforcing the breathing and relaxation techniques. Listen to them, focus on their voice and breathe with them. Do not focus on the pain, which is purely a by-product of the work your body needs to do in order to give birth. Instead, focus on helping your body do its job, bring in as much oxygen as you can by slowing your breathing and relaxing all those tense muscles.

The good news for those of you who will experience a back to back or occipito posterior labour is that the latent phase of labour is usually longer and more painful than the active phase. The mistake that most women make with these types of labour is taking their strong pain relief options in the latent phase of labour fearing that their active phase will be more painful.

It is important with this type of labour to use all those options of pain relief discussed earlier along with the other helpful methods. Back ache will be your primary complaint; however once you enter the active phase of labour, and your baby's head has turned, that back ache will ease greatly. If you do have a back to back labour and have managed without anything stronger than the methods mentioned earlier then you will now benefit. The large quantities of endorphins you produced are now working to lessen pain.

Your Environment

The environment for labour should closely mimic our ancestors' surroundings. There should be minimum distraction and the room should be as calming and relaxing as possible. The simplest way to achieve this is to ensure as few people as possible are around you in labour. You also need to keep any unnaturally light to a minimum, preferably with lights switched off, and music should be of the soothing variety, regardless of your normal listening taste. Aromatherapy is another excellent method of relieving stress and tension and lavender scented candles or wheat bags work extremely well.

Now is also a good time to switch the ringer on your telephone to silent and to resist the temptation of telling close friends and family that 'it's started'. The ensuing barrage of well-wishers will only disrupt this very delicate stage of your labour. This is the most finely balanced point of labour. The smallest distraction can slow it down or stop it all together.

That is not to say that if your labour does slow down or stop that something's gone wrong, it just means it is not *that time* yet. Just relax, don't overanalyse things and your labour should start again in its own time. If it is the middle of the night go to bed and try to sleep, if it is daylight try a gentle walk. During this time it is so important to minimise the production of stress hormones and maximise the production of oxytocin.

Overcoming Problems with your Labour

If your pregnancy has been normal and low risk there is no reason to assume that your labour and birth will be anything other than straightforward. This is especially true if your labour has started naturally and you have avoided strong forms of pain relief. In fact, the assumption should always be made that there will be no problem, that labour will progress without intervention and you will achieve a straightforward and normal birth. This should also be your default mind set, because why would there be a problem?

Unfortunately there are occasions when, even with the best of intentions, your labour slows down. This is known as dystocia and there are a number of options that can be used to reverse this:

- Change position, walk about or use the toilet.
- Nipple stimulation to increase oxytocin.
- It may be that the change of environment has led to the production of stress hormones, relax and wait thirty minutes.

If these methods fail the hospital staff, including your midwife or obstetrician, may discuss with you other means of increasing your contractions. These will include breaking your waters (known as artificial rupture of membranes) or the hormone drip, known as syntocinon. Providing there are no concerns regarding you or your baby it will be safe to use the non-intervention methods before consenting to having your waters broken or the hormone drip.

Another issue which may be encountered is a drop in your baby's heart rate. This does not always indicate a problem but may necessitate closer observation of your baby's heart beat with a heart rate trace known as a cardiotocograph or *C.T.G.* Likewise, your waters may break and show evidence that your baby has passed meconium. This in itself is not a problem but your midwife may want to ensure that your baby does not become distressed and recommend a continuous heart rate trace. Even with this you will still be able to stand. Your movement will be limited but you can ask to have it suspended to allow you to empty your bladder if needed.

Keeping Labour Going

Labour is a funny thing. It is unpredictable, can start without a second's notice and stop just as abruptly. In an effort to maintain contractions you may find that walking makes them more frequent and if this is the case then walk as much as you can. You may even find that sitting on the toilet makes them more intense. What you want to avoid is staying awake when the contractions are coming every thirty minutes. That is usually labour's way of telling you to go to bed and sleep or simply rest if you cannot.

On the subject of toilets they are extremely effective to use in labour if your baby is back to back. They work in a similar way to squatting by increasing the space in your pelvis. Using the toilet you are more likely to be able to maintain this position for longer than if squatting. This extra space allows your baby to move further down into your pelvis. Studies have shown that this position increases the room in your pelvis by 20-30 percent.

If your baby is in the back to back or occipito posterior, then the diameter of your baby's head as he tries to negotiate your pelvis is larger than if he was facing towards your spine. The anatomy of your pelvis makes it an elliptical shape at the top round in the middle and the opposite elliptical shape at the bottom. You then have your pelvic floor, a muscle which hangs like a sling from the bottom of your pelvis from front to back and side to side. This 'sling' forms a gutter shape which is higher at the back than the front. The purpose of this sling is to give resistance to the baby's head as he descends allowing him to make a quarter turn in the middle of your pelvis into the correct position to be born.

If your baby is back to back then his head is inclined to tip backwards making the diameter even larger. His head, now in a more awkward position is then forced down onto your pelvic floor in order to turn. As his head is slightly larger now this process of descending through the pelvis takes longer. The force of this process exerts greater pressure on the muscles and ligaments of the movable parts of your pelvis and that results in backache. If you do suffer backache, and back rubs don't relieve the pain, you may find that sitting on the toilet helps. This time on the toilet should give your baby's head enough room to descend onto the 'sling' of your pelvic floor and turn his head into the normal smaller diameter position.

Even if your baby is not back to back, by changing the shape and diameter of your pelvis you allow your baby's head to descend into your pelvis more quickly. As his head reaches your pelvic floor it will exert pressure, which initiates the 'Ferguson Reflex'. This reflex causes an increase in the production of oxytocin which in turn increases the strength, frequency and duration of the contractions.

There may be a temptation at this point to want to have a break from the contractions and adopt a position where they come less frequently and with less intensity. In order to reduce the amount of contractions your body needs to produce less oxytocin. The less oxytocin you produce the more likely it is that your labour will slow down or stop. In order to produce high levels of oxytocin try to maintain the position that gives you the most intense and frequent contractions and try other forms of pain relief. This will take effort and energy so it is important that you remember to feed your body to maximise its efficiency.

Eating & Drinking

While in labour your uterus, as a hard working muscle, is using up vast quantities of energy in the form of glucose. Your body can either use carbohydrates, which can be easily broken down with few waste products or it can convert fat stores. Breaking down fat stores is far less efficient at converting food into energy and produces a by-product called ketones and these ketones can slow down your contractions and with it your labour.

Because of this you should eat when you feel hungry and be encouraged to eat small amounts of food at meal times or to graze. Your gut will be much slower to empty in labour so you should avoid high fat foods and stick to bananas and toast as they are less likely to cause nausea and vomiting. If you do feel nauseous or unable to eat then glucose tablets are also effective at providing fuel for your body and reducing the production of ketones.

You should also keep well hydrated during labour as dehydration can cause problems with your baby's heart rate. Try to drink often and limit it to water if possible. Remember, if you are spending a lot of time in the bath you will still lose water through sweat.

By drinking adequate amounts of water your bladder will fill and obviously have less room. Although a full bladder rarely prevents your baby's head from descending through your pelvis the resultant trauma can cause bruising to the bladder muscle. This trauma and bruising may cause problems with passing urine after your baby's birth and is a common cause of stress incontinence in mothers. As you will be drinking more fluid than normal it is important to try to pass urine at least every four hours and attempt to do so every two hours. If your contractions have become sporadic and you are resting in bed then you do not need to wake to drink or pass urine.

Calling an Ambulance

If you do need to call an ambulance ask your partner to use their mobile phone as it allows them to perform tasks you may be instructed to do. If you're on your own then again, use your mobile phone if you can. Once you or your partner have made the call and given the relevant information to the staff quickly unlock your front door. If it is during daylight leave it slightly ajar, if it is during the night turn on all the lights on the bottom floor. Both will help to identify your home to the ambulance crew and allow them quick entry to your home. They will stay in contact with you until the ambulance crew arrives and even talk you through a birth if necessary.

Leaving for Hospital

So, you have decided that now is the right time to make your way to hospital. You will become stressed easily at this stage so you want to make sure that you keep your emotions in check. You can use breathing exercises discussed earlier to control your air intake and because you have your checklist ready you should not have to worry about anything. Your partner's job is to organise everything else, your only job is to stay focused and calm. Concentrate on your breathing and visualise your baby in your arms, your first breast feed or nappy change and try to avoid focusing on the contractions, which are merely your body's way of bringing your baby to you.

You will now see the benefits of having the checklist taped to the door from which you will exit the house. A quick check through the list and you are ready to go. Any upset at this point is unnecessary so your partner should make this transition as smooth as possible and should avoid asking too many questions of you. If you do find that there is a problem with your car simply come back inside your home and telephone for a taxi, or an ambulance if you're short on time. There really is no need to panic or worry, nothing is insurmountable if you and your birth partner are organised.

Summary checklist

Your Birth Environment

- Ensure there is minimal noise and disruption.
- Ensure that the lights are as dim as possible and preferably off.
- Use tranquil, soothing music.
- Use aromatherapy candles or wheat bags.
- Make yourself comfortable but preferably not in bed.
- Be on your own if you need to.

Keeping your Labour Going

- Adapt your environment appropriately –
  o Dim lighting.
  o Soft, tranquil music.
  o Minimal noise and distraction.
  o Aromatherapy.
- Use the position that gives you the most intense and frequent contractions.
- Avoid any position that reduces the frequency or intensity of your contractions such as lying down.
- Stay well hydrated and try to eat small amounts of easily digestible food.
- Reinforce to yourself that you are not a passenger in this labour, and that it is your body and you are in control.
- Empty your bladder regularly.

When to Contact your Midwife or Hospital

- If you think your waters have broken.
- If you notice fresh, red blood from your vagina (not to be confused with a 'show').
- If you feel your baby has not moved as much as normal.
- Any contractions before 37 weeks.
- Contractions coming every 3 minutes or more frequently.
- Contractions lasting for more than 1 minute.
- Constant abdominal pain.
- Difficulty in breathing.
- When you cannot cope with the pain any longer and have exhausted all methods of pain relief at home.
- If you feel pressure in your back passage similar to needing to poo and you feel like you *want* to push at the same time. (Not to be confused with *having* to push where you are unable to control the urge to push).

When to Call an Ambulance

- If you start pushing and have no control over it or have lost the ability to stop yourself from pushing. (This in itself is not an emergency but the quickest way of getting someone to you).
- Lots of blood coming from your vagina and bleeding down your legs (this is extremely rare).
- Severe difficulty in breathing, and/or chest pain.
- Constant abdominal pain with or without bleeding.

Chapter 10

Women with Complicated Pregnancies

You will hear, mostly from the media that more women are entering pregnancy with medical conditions. Depending on what these conditions are will determine whether your pregnancy and labour is classed as 'high risk'. Being in this category is not a slight on yourself but merely recognition that we're all different.

In most cases your condition will either have been long term or identified at some point in pregnancy. In each of these cases you will have seen an obstetrician for some of your antenatal appointments and your midwife for others. During your obstetric antenatal appointments you would have been given information about how this condition affects pregnancy and vice versa. This information will be purely to inform you of how to care for yourself and your baby during your pregnancy. If you are fortunate you may have been informed about the plans and procedures for your labour and this should help to prepare you for it. If not, your midwife should be able to tailor information about your care in labour to your specific condition.

Because of time constraints this is not always possible and you may find that your clinic appointments revolve around discussing your care in pregnancy and avoid your care in labour. For the most part little will change, but your consultant obstetrician may ask that you contact your midwife or labour ward at a particular time. She may ask that you inform them when you experience your first contractions or if your waters break. Each consultant obstetrician's advice will differ depending on which condition you have, so please do follow their advice. When you reach that predetermined time and contact your midwife or labour ward, remind them of the condition you have and the plan for your labour.

High Temperature in Labour

Not all conditions are detected in pregnancy and some will develop just before or during your labour. One of the most common of these is developing a high temperature in labour. There can be many reasons for this, such as an infection, an epidural or just as a response to labour.

Your temperature will be checked regularly in labour and if your midwife notices that it is beginning to rise she will check it more frequently. Your body's response to any rise in temperature is to make you feel warm so that you try to cool yourself down. You may ask for a fan or cool water and that usually suggests that you are able to prevent it from becoming too high. Your pulse rate may be raised so you may be encouraged to drink more water or be offered intravenous fluids and paracetamol may be used to reduce your body temperature.

These temperature reducing methods are offered because your baby will also experience the effects of your increased body temperature causing his heart rate to rise. Taking on fluid either by mouth or through a vein will help to reduce both your and his heart rates. If your temperature is below 37.5 degrees Celsius then you will not normally require investigations or treatment other than paracetamol and a cool environment. If your temperature is above 38 degrees Celsius it is unlikely to be a normal response to labour or epidural and more likely due to infection. You may experience this as shivering and feel cold, you may even request blankets. If you do then your midwife will take your temperature to check that your shivering is not 'rigors', your body's way of dealing with a high temperature. There is no immediate way of diagnosing an infection during labour. Your obstetrician will advise testing your blood and urine for bacteria. If you have suffered with a cough they may also want to test a sample of your sputum. They may then wish to start intravenous antibiotics and paracetamol if they have not already done so.

It is important not to treat women as high risk purely because they have had a slight rise in their body temperature. If your pregnancy was low risk prior to this, providing your baby is showing no signs of compromise, there would not usually be a re-assessment of your pregnancy to high risk. The only extra precautions will be more frequent checking of your temperature. If your temperature has increased and remained above 37.5 degrees Celsius then your obstetrician may wish to monitor your baby more closely using a heart rate trace. This should not prevent you from being as active and mobile as you wish.

Following the birth of your baby his temperature will be monitored along with his breathing and heart rate to look for signs of infection. Midwives will usually monitor him for around 24-36 hours on the postnatal ward. If there are signs that he may be developing an infection then the paediatricians will be asked to assess him and may wish to take some blood tests and give him antibiotics.

Although staying an extra few days in hospital may seem like an inconvenience there is good reason for your hospital and NICE guidelines advise this. Many babies will show no signs of infection during that time and be discharged home. For the handful of babies who may develop an infection they can become extremely ill very quickly and being closely monitored in hospital makes all the difference.

Pre-eclampsia

Although most conditions are picked up antenatally some may not develop until during labour or after birth. Pre-eclampsia is a case in point and the only treatment for it is delivery of your baby and placenta. It may be that you are being observed closely for this during pregnancy or that you are having your labour induced because of it. For some women though, the first they discover of this is when they are in labour.
Pre-eclampsia symptoms may include:
- High blood pressure.
- Protein in your urine.

- Headaches.
- Visual disturbances such as double or blurred vision.
- Pain under your ribs – epigastric pain.
- Swelling.
- Abnormal blood results.

Even with a healthy low risk pregnancy it is routine for your midwife to test your blood pressure and urine at your antenatal appointments. It is carried out to ensure that everyone is screened for this condition and during labour your blood pressure and urine are also regularly checked. For some women high blood pressure will simply be their body's response to stress and pain in labour and once they have relaxed it will return to normal. For others it may remain high and require treatment in the form of blood pressure medication to reduce it.

If your urine tests positive for protein at the same time as your blood pressure is high your midwife or obstetrician may want to perform blood tests to rule out pre-eclampsia. These results will also inform the anaesthetist if it is safe for you to have an epidural or spinal anaesthesia. In fact, you may be offered one as another method of reducing your blood pressure.

It may be that you have developed a mild form of this condition which effects up to ten percent of women. In a mild case, all that is necessary is to observe your blood pressure over the course of your labour and perhaps restrict the amount of fluid you drink. You may also be advised to have your baby monitored via a heart rate trace. Very rarely, in one to two percent of pregnancies women may develop a severe form or pre-eclampsia. They may become very unwell and require treatment with specialist drugs. In exceptionally rare cases it may also be necessary to perform a Caesarean section as an emergency to curtail labour and deliver your baby.

If you do develop the severe form of pre-eclampsia you will remain on the labour ward and under close observation for at least 24 hours. If you developed pre-eclampsia earlier in your pregnancy it may be that your baby needed to be born prematurely in order to treat your condition. If this is the case he will usually be cared for in the neonatal unit. He may be smaller than other babies his age due again to this condition and he may require closer observation.

Nothing can prevent pre-eclampsia, and nothing that you do causes it. It really is just one of these things and the only cure is delivery of your baby and placenta.

Obstetric Cholestasis

If you have been afflicted with severe itching in your pregnancy then your G.P. or midwife may have referred you to hospital for tests. During your assessment you will normally have had your baby monitored and also had blood tests. The itching in some cases is caused by a build-up of bile salts in your body, a condition known as obstetric cholestasis. This condition affects seven in one thousand pregnancies and it is more prevalent in women of Asian origin.

Normally bile salts flow from your liver to your gut to enable you to digest food. In this condition the bile salts become 'static' and don't flow properly causing a build-up. Blood test results determine whether you require medication

128

however the only cure for this is the birth of your baby. You may also be offered topical lotions such as calamine to ease the itching and will require regular blood tests during your pregnancy. There has been a suggested link to an increase in stillbirth with this condition and because of this your consultant obstetrician will usually offer to induce your labour after 37 weeks depending on the severity of the condition. The induction process for this condition is no different to any other. During labour your baby will be continuously monitored by a heart rate trace. Following birth the condition will clear up and your baby, if he is born at full term, will be cared for by you on the postnatal ward.

Diabetes

You could have been a diabetic since childhood, you may have developed the illness as an adult, or it may have only affected you since falling pregnant - gestational diabetes. There are signs in pregnancy that may point towards gestational diabetes and risk factors for developing the condition will be noted. Your hospital may have their own guidelines however NICE recommend offering glucose tolerance tests, where your blood is tested for levels of sugar to the following women:

- If your Body Mass Index is above 30 kg/m2.
- A previous baby weighing 4.5kg or more.
- A History of gestational diabetes.
- Family history of diabetes.
- Family origin with a high incidence of diabetes:
  o South Asian

- Black Caribbean
- Middle Eastern

Your care in pregnancy and labour will differ depending on whether you have gestational diabetes or pre pregnancy diabetes. Regardless of which you will be seen by obstetricians and midwives specialising in this area and their clinics may also include doctors specialising in diabetes. These multidisciplinary clinics ensure that your diabetes and your pregnancy are not treated as two separate conditions but that you as a person are treated as a whole. The clinics also eliminate the risks associated with the possible fragmentation of traditional care.

If you have had this condition prior to pregnancy then you will be aware of what your diet should and shouldn't include. As your body either does not produce enough insulin or your cells do not respond to it you need to be extremely careful balancing your intake of carbohydrates. Processed carbohydrates, such as white bread, is broken down quickly into simple sugars and without insulin to break this down it will cause the level of sugar in your blood to rise. Women in pregnancy are therefore advised to stick to a low glycaemic index (G.I.) diet and to take regular exercise.

Regular testing of your blood sugars throughout the day during pregnancy will inform your doctors whether additional medication is needed on top of diet to stabilise the condition. Doctors will devise a plan for your care in labour. If you are already using insulin in pregnancy then you will require an infusion of insulin in labour; If not then it may be that you will only have to measure your blood sugars regularly in labour.

If your blood sugars have been well controlled and your baby is normally grown you will usually be offered induction after 38 weeks' pregnancy. If your blood sugars are poorly controlled your baby may end up with a higher birth weight than he would naturally have had. This higher weight can cause problems when giving birth and therefore delivery by Caesarean section is more likely. If you have managed your gestational diabetes with diet and exercise you are more likely to have a smaller birth weight baby.

Your induction process will follow the same pathway as any other and your insulin use in pregnancy will determine whether or not you will require an insulin infusion in labour. Throughout labour your baby will be continuously monitored using a heart rate trace, although you should still be encouraged to be as mobile as possible. Following his birth your baby will have his blood sugars monitored to ensure that he is able to regulate his blood sugars at a normal rate. If he does not require treatment, only observation, then he should be able to remain with you on the postnatal ward.

If you have gestational diabetes then following the birth you shouldn't require any further treatment. You will however be offered follow up tests at around six weeks either in clinic or with your G.P. If you had diabetes before pregnancy then a plan for your postnatal treatment will have been arranged at your antenatal appointments.

Vaginal Birth After Caesarean Section

Reasons for a Caesarean section vary, however they are more likely to occur during labour for women in their first pregnancy. This is due to a number of factors, such as 'foetal distress' or 'dystocia of labour' where labour stalls completely. For others, Caesarean sections will be planned antenatally for reasons such as a breech position, placental problems or a previous Caesarean section.

Whatever the reason for a Caesarean section it is safe, in most cases, to plan for a vaginal birth in the next pregnancy. Your consultant obstetrician or consultant midwife will be able to discuss this with you further. If you gave birth by Caesarean section previously then your chance of having a vaginal birth next time is 70-90 percent. If you have had a vaginal birth previously as well as a Caesarean section then the probability increases to 90 percent.

The benefit of an elective Caesarean section is that you can plan when surgery will be and have some level of control over it. However, there is always the possibility that your labour could start before that date and you would then require an emergency Caesarean section.

Caesarean sections are not risk free and with each subsequent operation that risk rises. Because of scar tissue from a previous operation there is increased risk of bleeding, which may require a blood transfusion, and damage to internal organs, such as your bladder and bowel, can occur. As with any surgery the risk of developing blood clots also increases.

Additionally, your baby will not have experienced the stress of labour and due to this his lungs may not have fully initiated the transition to breathing. He may then go on to develop difficulty breathing which may require closer monitoring and treatment on the neonatal unit.

Having a scar on your uterus will also affect the area into which your baby implants. As your baby embeds into your uterus he is more likely to do this onto the lower part of your uterus and over your previous scar resulting in a placenta praevia. This condition will rule out the choice of a vaginal birth due to the potentially catastrophic blood loss that may occur whilst giving birth. If your placenta has implanted over your previous Caesarean section scar then the surgery itself also becomes extremely complicated. You may be required to attend the radiology department immediately prior to your surgery to limit the blood supply to your uterus. These factors should be considered if you are planning a large family.

By opting for a vaginal birth after a Caesarean section you are more likely to breastfeed successfully and the recovery time is also much quicker. To be successful with a vaginal birth after Caesarean section you need good support from birth partners and to remain as mobile as possible. Essentially you should aim to keep any intervention to a minimum as this will again reduce your chances of success.

The risks involved with a vaginal birth after Caesarean section are that for one in four hundred women the scar from their previous operation will open. This may then cause extreme blood loss for you, put your baby at risk and require an emergency Caesarean section. Vaginal births or Caesarean sections carry different risks and benefits but overall any risk is extremely small and either option is safe.

If you decide to opt for a vaginal birth after Caesarean section you can take measures to increase your chance of being successful. You may wish to avoid an epidural as it can slow down labour and make another Caesarean section more likely. There are plenty of techniques that you can use from earlier chapters and remember if you had an emergency Caesarean section before then this labour should be quicker. When you think that labour has started avoid the temptation of going into hospital too early. It is more likely to be a slower labour in hospital and you are more likely to use strong pain relief earlier. You should wait until your contractions are coming regularly - every five minutes and lasting for 60 seconds.

But you should inform your hospital if you have any of the following:

- Bleeding from your vagina.
- If your waters break.
- Any abdominal pain not connected to your contractions.
- Pain along the scar from your previous Caesarean section

Your midwife will assess your stage of labour by vaginal examination. This is important as it will give her a baseline to observe that your labour is progressing normally and not becoming too slow. A labour progressing slowly can be a sign things are not altogether normal and an intervention may be necessary at that stage. If you are in active labour she will also wish to commence a continuous heart trace to monitor your baby. You will normally have a cannula –a thin plastic tube - inserted in your hand and may have baseline bloods tests taken in case you require another Caesarean section. This will avoid any delay should this need to be done quickly.

Your baby also needs to be monitored in labour in case of signs that he is becoming distressed, which could indicate that your scar has opened. If this was the case you would require an emergency Caesarean section.

If labour is progressing more slowly than normal the hormone drip may be used to speed it up, however this will always be used with caution to prevent unnecessary pressure on your previous Caesarean section scar. However occasionally, your obstetrician may feel that the risks of starting the hormone drip are less than the risks of another Caesarean section.

Most hospitals, at present, do not offer water births to women who have had a previous Caesarean section as there is no clear evidence as to its safety in such cases. Many hospitals nowadays though have heart trace monitors that operate in water enabling you to have a water birth. If you are considering a water birth bear in mind that, although small there are still risks with a vaginal birth after Caesarean section.

It is more than likely that you will achieve a vaginal birth with minimal intervention. Once you have given birth, you will have the options of either a physiological or active management for delivering the placenta, providing you have avoided the hormone drip. Providing the rest of your labour ran smoothly and your baby is well, there is no stipulation on how long you should stay in hospital and for some women this may be as little as a few hours.

Chapter 11

What to Expect in Hospital

Entering a hospital environment, whether or not your pregnancy is regarded as high risk, may increase your anxiety levels. You have, after all, left the relative safety and serenity of your home and arrived into an alien, clinical place populated with midwives, doctors and support staff who spend much of their working life there. The hospital is an extension of their home life and as such you are seen as a visitor to that area. For many staff they will do their utmost to ensure that this transition from your home to hospital is as smooth as possible, indeed some go so far as to decorate and furnish rooms to give it a home from home feel. It is hoped the reduction in the clinical feel of the rooms will reduce the levels of stress hormones that you produce but it is inevitable that stress levels will rise and you may notice that your contractions become less frequent at this point.

If your pregnancy is high risk these less clinical rooms may not be available to you. But, in any case, you should be able to arrange the room and change the ambiance to reflect a more relaxing environment. The simplest way to do this is to move the bed to the side of the room, close the curtains, dim the lights and play soft music; your midwife should help you with this. Regardless of the complications you experience in your pregnancy and labour there are only extremely rare occasions where this change of use would be inappropriate.

The hospital bed is probably the greatest barrier to a normal birth; the use of it reduces the efficiency of your contractions and reduces the ability of your pelvis to expand to accommodate your baby through your birth canal. More importantly, women complain that their pain is greater when lying down.

As much as you are advised to avoid the bed there are occasions when a formal assessment of your progress in labour is necessary, especially if your labour has been classed as high risk. Your midwife may request that you lie down on the bed in order to carry out the assessment with accuracy but you should be able to leave the bed as soon as this has been done.

Examinations

Midwives use many skills to assess the stage of labour or the position the baby is in. Your midwife is able to predict the path that labour may take and advise on methods that can be used to help with the different types of labour. Abdominal palpation and vaginal examinations are key to these predictions. The abdominal palpation tells your midwife which way your baby is lying, for example, head down or breech. It also tells her how far down your baby's head is and whether he is back to back or facing your back. From this information and your behaviour, your midwife can determine how your labour may progress.

In hospital your labour care is led by you and the hospital's guidelines. It is usual practice for each hospital to have a guideline on care for each stage of labour and they are usually time limited. That is to say that once your cervix has opened, or dilated to a certain point you are deemed to be in 'active labour' and once in active labour there is guidance on how frequently and with what methods they will listen to your baby's heartbeat.

There is an expectation in active labour that your cervix will continue to dilate at a certain rate per hour and if progress falls short of this there are methods to increase the rate. The only way that the stage of labour can be established fully, and therefore set the clock ticking, is by performing a vaginal examination.

If you decline to have vaginal examinations your midwife will tailor your care to the stage of labour that she predicts you may be in and you will still be able to have the pain relief of your choice. Everyone's labour is different, some women need longer than others to give birth and some labours establish at a lesser or greater cervical dilatation than the standard. The benefit of avoiding vaginal examinations is that you allow your body to take as long as it needs to fully establish labour and give birth without a clock. The benefits of having a vaginal examination are that it gives you something tangible to focus on. Also, if your labour becomes high risk or complicated it will give the labour ward team more information and enable them to plan the appropriate care more thoroughly.

For example, if on palpation your midwife feels that your baby may be a breech presentation then she would wish to do a vaginal examination to determine what type of breech it is.

If your labour is straightforward and you feel that the contractions are not diminishing then vaginal examinations are merely a helpful tool for the midwife. If you feel that you would like to know where you are on the labour continuum or, if the labour ward staff are concerned in some way about your labour then a vaginal examination is extremely useful.

An abdominal palpation is the first procedure to be carried out and is exactly the same as the one that your community midwife did in pregnancy. You will then be asked to remove the clothing from your bottom half and bring your feet up towards your bottom then let your knees drop to the side. Your midwife or obstetrician will then insert two gelled fingers into your vagina to feel for your cervix. The procedure itself is sometimes uncomfortable but only takes a few moments and is not done during a contraction. If you need them to stop at any time simply tell them. After the vaginal examination they will tell you their findings and at what stage of the labour continuum you are on, and make a plan for your care in labour.

Stages of labour have many terms; early labour is also known as the latent phase of labour or '*not in established labour*' and active labour is also referred to as established labour. Regardless of the term used, if you are having contractions then you are by definition in labour. Whether your labour will continue or stop for a while will depend on which 'phase' of this stage of labour you are in: the '*active phase*' or the '*latent phase*'.

The early or latent phase of labour is defined by NICE as: "A period of time, not necessarily continuous, when there are painful contractions and there is some cervical change, including cervical effacement and dilatation up to 4cm".

The onset of active labour when there are: "Regular painful contractions and there is progressive cervical dilatation from 4cm." In other words your cervix reaching 4cm open is the defining moment for your labour, but only in the eyes of the midwives and obstetricians. To you it will feel no different to 3cm or 5cm open

For many women the latent phase of labour is a frustrating time. The contractions may last only a few hours before slowing abating and it may take days before they start again and for the same thing to happen. For other women the latent phase may last two or three days but the contractions never become more frequent than every twenty minutes. As you will be unaware of how long this phase of labour may last it is important that you eat and drink regularly and rest when you can.

A prolonged latent phase of labour is widely considered to be benign and not clinically significant so there is no need to be concerned provided you have an otherwise straightforward pregnancy and labour. As frustrating as this is please remember that the most effective environment for your labour, especially early labour is your home and this stage will last as long as it takes. Leaving your safe and calm environment during this phase and going to hospital will usually slow or stall your labour completely. Secondly, the hospital staff will only be able to offer you pain relief, of which only diamorphine and epidural are not able to be taken at home.

If you do attend hospital and find that you are in the latent phase of labour ask yourself '*do I really need to be here, would I be able to cope at home.*' If the answer is 'yes' and all is well with your labour then you are best to return home. If you feel that you need some pain relief ask if you may have some codeine to take home with you as some NHS Trusts offer this service. If you do decide to remain in hospital for the latent phase of your labour you will usually be admitted to an antenatal ward or remain on the assessment ward. Hospitals are very warm, dry environments so remember to keep drinking and try to find somewhere dark and secluded to reduce your stress hormones.

Bladder Care in Labour

Effective bladder care is extremely important in labour. Your bladder is a hollow muscular bag which stores urine and is capable of containing an average of between 400-600 millilitres of urine at any time. When stretched it sends a message to the brain that you need to pass urine. During pregnancy your bladder, due to its close proximity to your uterus, will be lifted out of your pelvis as your uterus grows. Your growing uterus will place added pressure on your bladder's capacity resulting in the sensation that you need to pass urine more frequently.

We all have a different capacity at which this will occur but it is on average 300 millilitres. Beyond this volume the sensation will increase and if left will result in pain in your lower abdomen. During labour you will already be experiencing lower abdominal pain so differentiating between bladder pain and contractions may be difficult.

Prolonged poor bladder care in labour can cause stress incontinence following the birth; to avoid this it is important to empty your bladder regularly during labour. If you find this difficult there is no need to worry as your midwife can advise you on good bladder care. It may be that you are dehydrated or if you are retaining urine there is the option of inserting a catheter to completely empty it. The advantage of a catheter is that it virtually eliminates problems associated with distending your bladder. You can either have a catheter passed which empties your bladder within a couple of minutes before it is removed or keep the catheter in until you're ready to push.

The disadvantages of having a catheter passed are risk of infection and discomfort; however you can request a numbing gel which will reduce the discomfort. Having a catheter inserted is a sterile procedure and you will be asked to adopt the same position as you would for a vaginal examination. The procedure only takes a few moments and is only mildly uncomfortable.

Once your midwife has completed the procedure there should be no limit to your mobility unless your baby is being monitored by a heart rate trace.

Monitoring Your Baby's Heartbeat

Your midwife will have listened to your baby's hear rate initially and as you enter the active phase of your labour she will do this more frequently. Monitoring your baby's heartbeat is to assess whether or not your baby is coping with the rigors of labour. The midwife will use a handheld 'Doppler' in most cases similar to the one used in your antenatal clinic appointments. This allows the midwife to take a snapshot of how your baby is coping at that point. The heart rate will not confirm whether or not your baby is coping with labour but as your labour is low risk the assumption is that he will be. Most healthy babies, who are coping well with their labour, will drop their heart rate during a contraction. This is normal and not a concern.

To be classed as low risk an assessment will have been done by your community midwife antenatally. She will consider your medical history and previous pregnancies and births. Using all the information and hospital guidelines she will gauge the level of risk of your baby becoming distressed during labour. If you are classed as 'high risk' you will be offered a continuous heart rate trace. This is because the risks of your baby becoming distressed in labour are higher and as such he needs to be more closely monitored to pick up any distress promptly. This is especially important in babies with meconium in their waters when they break.

Cardiotocograph (CTG)

Occasionally labour does not follow a normal, low risk path and for these eventualities it may be necessary to monitor your baby's heart rate more closely. The current NICE guideline only recommends heart rate traces for complicated or high risk labour. That may sound strange but the heart rate trace has a high false positive rate of around 60 percent. This means that in six out of ten women the heart rate trace will interpret heart rate changes as indicative of distress when there is none. If you have been classed as 'low risk' then the risk of your baby becoming distressed is extremely low. In view of the fact that heart rate trace has such a high false positive rate, using this method in low risk women would create unnecessary intervention and the risks of that intervention are not outweighed by the benefits to you or your baby.

If you are classed as 'high risk' there will be a higher rate of distressed babies and using the hand held doppler method does not allow for frequent enough checks of a baby's heartbeat. Although there is a high false positive rate it is more likely, being in the high risk group, that this will be a true positive indicator of distress.

Heart rate trace is reliable. It has a high negative predictive value and by that it is meant that when classed as 'normal' it demonstrates that 98 babies out of 100 are not distressed. This statistic is both reassuring for yourselves and for your midwives and obstetricians. If you are classed as low risk and have anxiety surrounding your baby's wellbeing throughout labour you may wish to request a continuous heart rate trace. Although not recommended for low risk labour it may alleviate your fears knowing that if the heart rate trace is normal then your baby is probably well.

Do bear in mind that all babies need to be stressed during labour. During labour babies will exhibit stress in different ways. The majority of babies will drop their heart beat during a contraction in response to the sudden restriction of blood flow to the placenta at that time. This pattern of 'decelerations' in the heart rate is not suggestive of distress unless they are accompanied with other changes to your baby's heartbeat, such as if the overall heart rate has risen or the difference in the overall heart rate, known as variability, in one minute has reduced.

Remember though, six in ten babies will show signs of distress when there is none. Therefore, rather than reassuring you that your baby is well a continuous heart trace in low risk labour may only increase your anxiety. This is because once the heart trace shows decelerations, or a drop in the heart rate midwives and obstetricians become more vigilant of that heart trace. This vigilance will require other members of staff to also assess the heart trace and that it not ideal for your labour environment.

In high risk labour, where there are real concerns that a baby may not cope with labour, then a heart trace offers reassurance of his wellbeing at the expense of possibly requiring invasive testing. The heart trace can be used in any position but your movement may be limited by the length of the leads that attach to the machine.

Your baby's heart rate is obtained by placing an ultrasound transducer on your abdomen over his heartbeat. Another sensor is placed at the top of you abdomen to monitor contractions and bands are then attached around your abdomen to keep them in place. Both your contractions and your baby's heartbeat are traced at simultaneously either onto paper or stored electronically. The trace is constantly assessed by your midwife and periodically she may ask another member of staff for a second opinion or a fresh pair of eyes.

Occasionally your baby's heartbeat may be difficult to pick up over your abdomen. Sometimes this is due to you or your baby's position or it may be due to the distribution of fat in your abdomen. When the heartbeat is not detected the heart trace will no longer have a solid line along the heartbeat but portions of it missing. This is known as 'loss of contact'. When this occurs your midwife will ask herself the question, *"Do I need this information"*. More often than not the information is needed and your midwife will then discuss with you a 'Foetal Scalp Electrode (FSE)' also known as a 'clip'. This 'clip' or FSE is attached to your baby's scalp by the midwife whilst performing a vaginal examination. The clip will provide greater information of the frequency of your baby's heartbeat and resolve the problem of loss of contact. Having it applied will also allow the belt and transducer at the bottom of your abdomen to be removed and allow you greater mobility in labour.

Although it sounds extremely invasive for your baby the clip is tiny and sits on his first layer of skin. He will not feel anything and it does not put him at a greater risk. If this method is being advised then it is done so with you and your baby's best interests foremost in mind. If he is showing signs of distress then this method will give more information.

Foetal Blood Sampling

To find out whether your baby is distressed a blood test or Foetal Blood Sample (FBS) is usually taken. To carry out this test you will be asked to move onto your left side and your right leg will be raised using a wedge or lithotomy rest. In this position your midwife or obstetrician will gently insert a plastic or metal tube into your vagina. A light on the end will allow them to see your baby's head and they will then make a small nick on the top of his head and take a tiny sample of blood to be tested. It is usual practice to take three samples and they will act on the lowest reading. From taking the sample from baby's head to getting a result takes around ten minutes.

The blood is tested for levels of oxygen and acid, a process which takes around three minutes. This blood test is a very good indicator of how your baby is coping in labour and how he is likely to cope. The disadvantage of this test is that it can be uncomfortable for you and may have to be performed more than once during labour. As explained earlier, a heart rate trace picks up problems when six times out of ten there are none. If obstetricians were to carry out Caesarean sections based on that information then many would be done unnecessarily. NICE advises that heart rate trace monitoring should only be carried out if the hospital has the facilities to conduct foetal blood sampling. This is because the FBS test can very accurately detect 'foetal hypoxia' and 'acidaemia'.

As your blood flows to your placenta the oxygen and other nutrients it carries are transferred through the placenta into your baby's blood supply. In turn your baby then deposits his waste products in his blood such, as carbon dioxide, back into your placenta and from there your circulation. If he becomes distressed he will build up more carbon dioxide in his blood and by-products such as hydrogen ions. The hydrogen makes your baby's blood acidic hence the reason why a pH or 'acid test' is carried out. A neutral pH of seven is neither acidic, like the hydrochloric acid in our stomachs, nor alkaline like bleach. Water has a pH of seven.

Hydrogen ion build up is normally prevented by buffers in your baby's blood which mop up the molecules and maintain a neutral pH level. Babies can usually cope and keep on top of this hydrogen clean-up, however, if they are not receiving enough oxygen they begin to build up carbon dioxide levels and the by-product of that, hydrogen. These levels increase until eventually the buffers that mop up the hydrogen, preventing his blood from becoming acidic, are spent.

Testing the pH of babies' blood allows labour ward staff to judge the safest time for delivery. Too early and you may end up with an unnecessary Caesarean section, too late and he will need resuscitated. The standard point is a pH reading below 7.20. If your midwife or obstetrician becomes concerned that your baby's heart rate trace may be showing evidence of distress they will ask permission to perform a foetal blood sample.

If the results are above pH 7.25 then the test may be repeated in one hour. If the results are pH 7.20 to 7.24 then this is classed as borderline and the test would normally be performed within thirty minutes if you have not given birth. A pH result of below 7.20 is indicative of foetal distress and will require a Category I Caesarean section. This is discussed in a later chapter, 'Caesarean Section in Labour'. Although the thought of this may be frightening, because your baby was monitored so closely he will usually be delivered at the optimal time.

Bleeding in Labour

There are many reasons why you may bleed in pregnancy but it is relatively uncommon, affecting only three to five women in one hundred. Around 40 percent will bleed for no identifiable reason, but it is more common in women who have given birth before. The most common cause is the action of labour itself and it is very rare that bleeding in labour is anything more sinister than this.

Following a vaginal examination or membrane sweep you will find that you pass what is known as a heavy 'show'. This is heavier blood loss than you would have noticed when your show was passed at home, but it is still just a show. Your midwife will reassure you that this is to be expected following an examination and providing the bleeding settles no further action will be needed.

More rarely, if you notice blood loss that is fresh and red then it is unlikely to be classed as a 'show' and will probably require further investigation. Again, this will depend on whether or not you have pain, whether your labour was low risk and what stage of labour you are in. If your labour was low risk and you have no pain with the bleeding then your midwife will normally commence you on a heart trace to monitor your baby. This bleeding may be a sign that your placenta is coming away early from your uterus. If this happens then there may be a reduction in the amount of blood that your baby receives and as a result he may show signs of distress. Equally, he may not show any signs of distress and will cope well with labour and birth. Observing him for signs of distress using a heart rate trace means you are able to achieve a normal birth rather than having a Caesarean section or assisted birth as a precaution.

If you do experience bleeding from your vagina in labour your midwife will ask your consent to place a cannula (thin plastic tube) into the back of your hand. This will allow her to compensate for any blood loss by introducing fluids intravenously into your blood stream.

If you had a previous Caesarean section and wish a vaginal birth then the medical staff will be slightly more concerned if you begin to pass blood from your vagina. The severity of the bleeding and whether it is accompanied with any pain will determine whether your obstetrician advises a repeat Caesarean section. Whilst pushing you may also notice vaginal bleeding; it is usually caused by the slight trauma of baby descending and it nothing to worry about. His chin or nose can cause this and it is more usual in back to back babies when they begin to turn and nothing to worry about.

An extremely rare cause of bleeding is placental abruption, where the placental lining separates from the uterus, and is accompanied by constant abdominal pain. In such a case the obstetrician will either carry out a Caesarean section or assisted birth with your consent. This decision is dependent on the stage of labour you are in and how the blood loss has affected your baby.

Chapter 12

Having your Labour Induced

Induction of labour is defined as the use of artificial means to bring on birth. Synthetic hormones prepare your cervix and stimulate uterine contractions. Your membranes will, in most cases, need to be broken to maximise the effects of the artificial hormone syntocinon although your membranes may rupture of their own accord and this may establish labour without the need for hormone drip.

There are many well-meaning people who recount horror stories of labour and even more with terrible tales of induced labour. It is not the induction process that is troubling to women but the length of time it takes. Leave anyone on their own for long enough and they will over analyse any situation. The lack of sleep women are also faced with may contribute to this emotional state. By keeping your mind occupied and avoiding fixating on potential problems will help the drugs given to you induce your labour rather than hinder then. If you have dwelt on the possible pitfalls of labour you will become anxious, produce adrenalin and cortisol and limit the amount of oxytocin your body produces.

Remember the balance of oxytocin and endorphins? These natural pain killers are thought to be 500 times stronger than morphine.

The coping strategies that you would use in an induced labour are no different from those used in a spontaneous labour. You should still be able to remain upright and mobile as both the heart trace and hormone drip will allow this. It may be that the induction process itself may have affected your ability to use your coping methods effectively. If you do feel that you need strong pain relief then use it. Epidurals and opiates are excellent forms of pain relief and should not be denied to you, neither should you deny them to yourself if you feel you need them.

NICE guidance on induction of labour is followed by most hospitals in the United Kingdom although their timings of this and indications for it may vary slightly from consultant to consultant.

Reasons for Induction of Labour

The most common reason for induction of labour is being 'post mature' or 42 weeks' gestation however different hospitals have different criteria for induction dates.

Inducing labour before 42 weeks is to prevent complications associated with ageing of the placenta. This aging is caused by a build-up of calcium in the placenta; a process which begins at around 40 weeks' gestation. The build-up limits the blood flow and can cause 'placental insufficiency'. There is no set time when this will occur, it is just an average and your ethnic background will also have bearing on when this may occur. However, the risk of stillbirth rises sharply at 43 weeks.

Your decision should always balance the risks of induction versus the risks of not being induced. You may decide not to be induced at 42 weeks. Ultrasound scans and heart rate monitoring of your baby will inform you how he's coping inside. NICE, based on clinical evidence, has balanced the risks and advises induction of labour at no later than 42 weeks.

Some consultant obstetricians offer induction of labour at 40 weeks in the case of women over 40 years old in their first pregnancy, and those pregnant through invitro fertilisation (IVF). You may also be offered induction of labour at around 38 weeks' gestation if you have diabetes or obstetric cholestasis, although this would depend on how well controlled your condition is. Your consultant obstetrician will be able to discuss this with you further.

For twin pregnancies 37 weeks' gestation is considered term and your consultant obstetrician will usually offer to induce your labour at that time. You will have your date for induction booked which will enable you to prepare beforehand. There are however situations where you may be offered induction of labour straightaway. These include:

- If your baby has persistently moved less than previously and you have been monitored for this.
- If you have suffered from recurrent bleeds from your vagina.
- If you have high blood pressure and significant protein in your urine.

- If an ultrasound scan has detected a concern or problem.
- If your waters have broken and you have not gone into spontaneous labour.

It may be that rather than being admitted immediately for induction of labour you are given a membrane sweep. This is advised at around 40 weeks as it increases the likelihood that you will begin to labour spontaneously and reduces the need for induction of labour. If this is unsuccessful your midwife can then make an appointment for your labour to be induced if you wished.

What does Induction of Labour Involve?

Firstly, your midwife will perform a vaginal examination to determine whether or not she can break your waters. If she cannot and she determines that your cervix needs to be 'ripened', then she will insert a prostaglandin pessary or gel into your vagina. Prostaglandin is a hormone that will soften your cervix and is delivered topically to the cervix and comes in either tablet form, in a gel or as a tampon. The length of time each of these methods takes differs and each have their own benefits.

The tampon method has the advantage of working for 24 hours without needing repeated vaginal examinations. The gel and tablets require further applications every six hours to a maximum of three times.

Before this takes place your baby's heart rate will be checked using a heart rate trace to confirm that he is not stressed. Providing you do not experience any pain or contractions during that time and your baby's heart rate is normal, the heart trace will be removed. If you do experience contractions at any point during this process then the heart rate trace will recommence to ensure he has not become distressed in the intervening period. Although you will normally have his heartbeat listened to periodically throughout this time some hospitals do encourage women to go home at this point and return at a predetermined time.

You will usually experience 'prostin pains', which are similar to period pains and your midwife will be able to discuss all your pain relief options with you. On a positive note, if you experience any sensations in your lower abdomen, it is a sign that the hormone is working.

After a given time your midwife will perform another vaginal examination to see if your waters are ready to be broken. If this is possible then she will either break them there and then or move you to a labour room.

This process does not always work first time. In some cases the obstetrician will offer delivery of your baby by Caesarean section and others will either repeat the process straightaway or rest you for a period of time before retrying. You will always be included in the discussions and you should be encouraged to ask questions, especially if you do not agree with their plan of care.

Once your waters are broken and your midwife has no concerns about your baby then you will be able to mobilise. This will encourage your baby's head to press on your cervix and hopefully start your labour naturally. Because of the

155

benefits of this method you will normally be given around two to four hours during which time your midwife will be checking on you and your baby. If you are able to avoid the hormone drip, depending on your reason for induction, continuous monitoring of your baby by a heart rate trace may not be necessary. From this point it is hoped that your labour would follow the path of any natural labour and that pain relief and intervention will be minimal.

However, if the hormone drip is needed you will be commenced on a heart rate trace to ensure that your baby is not stressed. A cannula will then be inserted into the back of your hand and through this the hormone drip will pumped. The dosage is gradually increased whilst you are as mobile as possible, changing positions regularly. Eventually, you will notice that tightenings in your abdomen become stronger and develop into contractions. This is no different than normal spontaneous labour so focus on your breathing and ensure that your birth partner is helping you with your coping techniques. If you do find that you are struggling to cope with the intensity of the contractions and feel you need pain relief ask your midwife to examine your cervix. It may be that you are nearing the end of your labour and are in transition.

Risks of Inducing Labour

If you are using the hormone drip your baby's heart rate will be continuously monitored by a heart rate trace. Every labour is different. For some women their uterus will contract frequently and for others, less so. By using a hormone drip the frequency of your contractions and how baby is coping with them will be determined by your obstetrician. NICE and the Royal College of Obstetricians and Gynaecologists recommends no more than five contractions in ten minutes and fewer if signs show baby is becoming distressed.

As some babies require fewer contractions to be born it may be that those babies will not cope with the standard frequency associated with the hormone drip. They may exhibit signs that they are struggling and further testing using foetal blood sampling may be required to ensure that they have not become distressed.

There is an increased risk of foetal distress with induction of labour and therefore the need for a Caesarean section is increased. Also, because women are more likely to opt for strong pain relief there is also an increase in assisted births.

The hormone drip must be used with caution in women who have had a previous Caesarean section or have had more than one child. This is due to the very small risk that their uterus may rupture or their scar open and it is for these reasons that the benefits of induction of labour should outweigh the risks. It is also why most consultant obstetricians no longer offer induction of labour at maternal request even in the presence of symphysis pubis dysfunction (severe pelvic pain) or previous quick labours.

For most women, induction of labour is not the experience they were expecting and that is largely due to a lack of information. When women do search for that information it is invariably on the internet where many myths and untruths surrounding induction of labour exist. The NICE website offers all the information you should need on induction of labour.

Chapter 13

Helping to Reduce Anxiety & Pain

Whether you have a spontaneous labour or need to be induced you will experience anxiety. The more anxious you become the more pain you appear to feel, it's called the 'fear-pain cycle'. If you can manage your levels of anxiety then you should be able to cope with your labour pain more effectively. Everyone tolerates different levels of pain and anxiety and there are many forms of pain control available to use.

An amazing thing about labour and birth is the way women will instinctively behave, as if they have all read the same textbook. Their behaviour is so similar that experienced midwives are able to pinpoint their stage of labour.

Women who become fearful or who have little in the way of emotional support tend to be those who will request pain relief. Those women who have good emotional support and are prepared for labour without fear will use little or no pain relief.

Water Blisters

Back to back labours can cause tremendous back ache and water blisters is an effective method of relieving this pain. However, it is a relatively new practice and not many midwives will be able to provide this service. This technique has been used for more than 25 years by midwives in Scandinavian countries and research has shown that water is as effective, if not more so, than local anaesthetic.

In labour the sacral dimples or 'Rhombus of Michaelis' become pronounced and your partner will notice them as a diamond shape on your lower back. Small amounts of water are injected just under the skin at the four corners of the rhombus. It offers pain relief for up to sixty minutes on average, however women do report that injection of the water is uncomfortable.

Codeine

Codeine is a pain relief usually used in the early stages of labour. It is often used in conjunction with paracetamol as this helps your body maximise its effects. It is an opiate of the same family as morphine and is also a restricted drug. Codeine is given in tablet form, either on its own, with paracetamol or as one tablet also containing paracetamol known as co-codamol. However, studies show separate tablets are more effective.

As with all opiates codeine causes constipation. After having your baby you may need a stool softener. Other side effects include drowsiness, nausea and vomiting which can all be treated. Codeine provides pain relief for two and a half to three hours however be aware that the drowsiness you experience can also affect your baby.

Entonox

Entonox (known as gas and air) is an extremely effective form of pain relief, especially in the latter stages of labour. Entonox is inhaled and has the benefit of being usable during a water birth. It comes in cylinders or through a main hospital supply which is attached through the wall. The main benefits of entonox are its ease of use and the speed at which you will notice its effect. Because it is already 'active' meaning that your body does not need to do anything with it, it has its peak action 30 seconds after using it. It is also exhaled in the same state so its effects are out of your system in around 60 seconds. As it takes 30 seconds to become effective it should be used as soon as you feel the first flutter of your contraction and stopped when the sensation subsides.

Topical Local Anaesthetic

An anaesthetic cream or gel is applied to the skin and given a few moments to work. They are used primarily as 'instillagel' when having a catheter sited and besides numbing the area they have antibacterial qualities. 'Emla' cream is applied to the skin prior to an injection and is effective for women who fear injections but want pain relief.

Epidural

An epidural will completely remove pain. The medication is administered through a thin plastic tube inserted into your lower back by an anaesthetist. You will be required to stay very still during most of the procedure and will be sat upright on the bed facing your partner.

The anaesthetist uses sterile equipment, so it is important not to touch anything. The procedure takes an average of 15 minutes and you should feel it starting to work after around 20 minutes. Once it has been sited it will be taped down and attached to a pump which will deliver a set amount of pain killing drug continuously; it will not run out. You will then sit upright to ensure that the medication is evenly distributed and your midwife will begin monitoring your blood pressure and your baby's heart rate.

Occasionally the medication can cause your blood pressure to drop and if this happens you will be laid flat and moved onto your left hand side. You will be given fluid into a needle in the back of your hand and after a few minutes your blood pressure should normalise. During that time it is usual for your baby's heart rate to drop and this should also recover before six minutes.

For one in ten women the epidural is ineffective or only partially so. In such cases a higher dose of medication is given or the anaesthetist will move or reinsert the plastic tube.

Whilst the epidural is working your midwife will keep a close eye on your blood pressure and monitor your baby's heart rate. However, if your labour is still classed as low risk you won't normally require a continuous heart rate trace.

Some labour wards offer mobile epidurals whilst others believe, that in order to have a proper effect, higher doses are required, which leaves you less mobile and do not offer them as an option for pain relief. Disadvantages of an epidural include a higher rate of assisted birth, such as forceps or ventouse birth. This is because an epidural slackens the pelvic floor, makes it hard for a woman to know when to push and because mums to be are lying down in bed to push. You may also develop a severe headache after the procedure.

In an effort to reduce the side effects associated with epidurals and pushing, some midwives may offer to stop the epidural before you begin to push, allowing you more sensation of where to push.

Regardless of these factors, whether you choose to use epidural is up to you and no one should influence that decision.

Diamorphine

This is the generic name for heroin and is an effective form of pain relief although it is technically a sedative. It is given by injection into a muscle or, as morphine, into a vein. Its side effects include sedation, nausea, vomiting and respiratory depression (your breathing becomes less frequent and efficient). It also crosses over the placenta and into your baby's circulation and consequently your baby may be born sleepy, his feeding may be effected and he may need help with his initial breathing. If you plan to breastfeed following diamorphine in labour you would normally be advised to wake your baby regularly to feed in the initial 24 hours following his birth.

Pethidine

Pethidine is a synthetic form of injectable pain relief and has similar pain relieving effects as morphine. It has more side effects, but they are shorter lasting and these side effects include nausea, vomiting, dizziness, sedation and respiratory depression.

No Place Like Home

Midwives have long held the belief that with right environment women have the ability to labour and birth without any intervention or pain relief. In fact many Midwifery Led Units are modelled around a home from home environment.

We cannot escape that home is the best environment to labour in. It is where you feel safe and secure and you have access to all your home comforts. It is also the place where you are in control and any member of staff would be a guest in your home. You then have to leave this warm, safe environment where your body is attuned to your surroundings and enter a very noisy, cluttered and clinical environment. You have a natural urge to return to your home.

When you arrive in hospital you will notice that your contractions are less frequent and lack the same intensity. You will also realise that they have slowly diminished since you left home. On arrival at hospital your midwife will ask you how often your contractions were coming or how far apart they were. It is now you will realise that they are probably half as frequent as they were and no longer require the pain relief that brought you in. Don't worry, this is a normal response, in fact it may benefit you that your contractions are no longer so strong, or that you no longer want pain relief.

When you do finally arrive in your room you should reorganise it. The bed should be moved to the side of the room or removed from the room if the room is small. If the bed remains in the room you can raise it to your chest level and lean over it and if you begin to feel tired you can ask your partner to sit on the bed whilst you sit on a chair or birthing ball facing him. You can then lean forwards and rest your head on his knee.

The room lights should also be dimmed and if there is no facility in the room to dim the lights ask the midwife to switch them off and ask your birth partner to play your music or birth hypnosis CD. If you have taken aromatherapy essential oils with you use them now; you can either apply them as an atomiser or by an electric oil burner. The most effective oils to use at this point will be a mixture of lavender and clary sage as those are relaxing and encourage the production of oxytocin.

Your birth partner can help build your nest environment and offer gentle words of encouragement, water, provide soothing massages and pain relieving back rubs. Your midwife will remain at a respectful distance and be as unobtrusive as possible as she listens to your baby's heartbeat and will offer advice on positions and help you cope as your contractions begin to pick up.

Over the following 30 to 60 minutes you should relax into your new surroundings and the adrenalin and other stress hormones that were coursing through your body will diminish. As these stress hormones reduce you can encourage your body to produce oxytocin; there are a number of ways to do this. You can roll your nipples between your thumb and forefinger, you can roll your hips or more simply, cuddle your partner. You should now feel almost as relaxed and safe as you did at home and unsurprisingly your midwife will also feel the calming effect of you environment. The dim lighting and soft music will encourage her to talk quietly and not unnecessarily. Any necessary visitors to your room will also be encouraged to keep a respectful silence.

The more effective the environment the quicker you will produce adequate amounts of oxytocin, so remain calm and go back to coping techniques from earlier in labour at home. Remember your breathing techniques.

Because you are in active labour cervix will be opening and it may be that it has opened more quickly than you imagine. It is not uncommon for women's cervix to open 8cm in ten minutes whether it is their first or forth baby.

With this in mind, before you decide on pain relief it is worthwhile giving your body time to produce more quantities of endorphins to combat the pain. Just like oxytocin, endorphins have to work into your system, so be patient, your contractions will then return to similar levels as before. Change position regularly during that time and try to focus on breathing and relaxing your shoulder and neck muscles. Think of your new baby and his first feed, the colour of his hair. Think of the first time you take him outside to meet the world or introduce him to the rest of his family.

Waiting for your natural pain killers to become effective will not take long but if you focus and fixate on the pain it will seem like an age. Don't bottle up fears or concerns and tell your midwife, she's there to help.

Chapter 14

Waters Breaking

Your waters can break by themselves (known as a spontaneous rupture of membranes) or are broken for you (known as artificial rupture of membranes). Once the waters break there is no longer a soft cushion between your baby's head and your cervix. This pressure exerted by your baby's head on your cervix stimulates the production of prostaglandins and these prostaglandins cause softening or 'ripening' of your cervix.

Oxytocin is also produced causing the muscles of your uterus to contract and constant agitation of your cervix by your baby in labour ensures a steady production of oxytocin and prostaglandin. By removing pressure from your cervix you reduce this production which is why lying in bed for long periods in labour should be avoided.

It may not always be possible for your baby's head to cause pressure on your cervix. In some cases his head may still be high in your pelvis or in an awkward position, such as back to back. With less pressure on your cervix you are less likely to have contractions and labour spontaneously. A hindwater rupture, where the membranes break above your baby's head can leave a cushioned membrane of water still below his head preventing that much needed pressure on your cervix.

Occasionally your water may break before you have any contraction and as these membranes were protecting your baby from the risk of infection your midwife may discuss commencing the hormone drip to artificially induce contractions immediately or once 24 hours has elapsed. With the possibility that the membranes in front of your baby's head may still be present a forewater artificial rupture of membranes may be discussed with you. By breaking your waters the soft cushion that is preventing your baby's head exerting sufficient pressure on your cervix and help you to labour without the hormone drip.

Occasionally in labour your contractions may stall and your labour stutter to a halt or your cervix may not be opening to the extent that is expected for labour, after exhausting all other methods of increasing oxytocin production, your midwife may offer to break your waters. This is usually a very effective method of getting your labour back on track by increasing the frequency and strength of your contractions but studies have shown that it will only speed up labour by around 20 minutes.

To break your waters your midwife will first palpate your abdomen to ensure your baby's is head down or 'cephalic'. You then lie down in the same position as you would for a vaginal examination. Wearing gloves and using gel she will insert two fingers into your vagina and locate your cervix. She may need to gently open your cervix and move it forward in order to make the procedure simpler. She then introduces a thin plastic rod, similar to a crochet hook, into your vagina running it along the inside of her hand. Once the tip of the rod is against the tip of her fingers she will turn the rod so that the small sharp tip rests against your membranes. With her two fingers resting against the rod she will then apply gentle pressure to break the waters.

You will be aware of pressure and will feel warm fluid draining from your vagina. Once this occurs your midwife will remove her fingers from your vagina and listen to your baby's heartbeat. You will then be encouraged to stand, sit upright or go for a walk. Whether or not you will need to have a continuous heart trace following the procedure will depend on the colour of the fluid that comes away and how your baby has responded to the procedure.

Very occasionally, breaking your waters causes baby to rapidly descend through the pelvis, resulting in the baby's heartbeat dropping. This only lasts three or four minutes, during which time your midwife will move you onto your side and may call for assistance. She will continue to reassure you and your partner and answer any questions you may have.

Group B Streptococcus Infection

An infection of concern to midwives, obstetricians and paediatricians is called Group B Streptococcus or' Group B Strep'. Group B Strep is a bacterium found in your vagina and gut which is present in up to a third of the population and it is transient, meaning it may not always be present throughout your pregnancy. We all have colonies of different bacteria in our digestive tracts, throats, skin, etcetera, and most of the time they do not make us ill.

Confusion exists around Group B Strep with many couples anxious about the safest course of action. Currently in the U.K. women are not routinely screened for this infection because it is transient although women will be offered a test for the infection if they present with a vaginal discharge or threatened premature labour. The swabs take 48 hours to grow the bacteria and if the Group B Strep is identified then antibiotics are offered in labour to protection the baby. Use of antibiotics is not risk free, and the greatest risk is that you become sensitive or allergic to them and they can also cause nausea and diarrhoea.

Around 50 percent of babies born to mothers carrying Group B Strep will pick up the bacteria and be colonised by it. About one to two percent of that group will go on to develop severe Group B Strep infection, either as early onset (before two days old) or late onset (after two days old). Even with medical care ten percent of those babies that develop a severe infection will die. This severe infection or 'sepsis' is most likely to occur in babies who are premature and where there has been prolonged rupture of membranes, usually longer than 24 hours.

With sepsis being a real danger to new born babies you may wonder why every woman is not given antibiotics, regardless of whether the swab is positive or negative. In the USA screening for and treatment of Group B Strep is routine and they greatly reduced their Group B Strep infection rate in newborns. However, the number of babies dying of infections remained constant because other infectious bacteria took hold. Antibiotics merely removed one bacterium leaving a vacuum for another.

Current NICE guidance is to limit antibiotic use and hospitals have differing guidelines on the management of Group B Strep however routine screening of all women for Group B Strep is not recommended, only those that are in a risk group.

NICE recommend intravenous antibiotic cover continuously throughout labour if you have had a positive Group B Strep swab result in this pregnancy or have previously had a baby infected with Group B Strep. If you wish to be tested for Group B Strep and do not fall into a risk group you can get it done privately through your family doctor. Or there is a postal service which can be found on the Group B Strep Support website. The test should ideally be carried out between 35-37 weeks of pregnancy.

If you do test positive for Group B Strep the antibiotic of choice is benzylpenicillin and there is an alternative for those allergic to penicillin. Both are given through a needle in your hand every four hours during labour and providing you've had at least two doses of the antibiotic during your labour paediatricians will usually monitor your baby for signs of infection over a few days. If you gave birth before getting two doses paediatricians may advise that baby has intravenous antibiotics. The antibiotics are very effective at combatting Group B Strep and the risk of your baby developing this infection drops from one in three hundred to less than one in six thousand.

Chapter 15

Caesarean Section

Most women in labour, whether high or low risk will achieve a vaginal birth and for a high proportion it will be a normal birth. Natural birth rates differ greatly between hospitals; some with below and others with above average assisted birth rates. Caesarean section rates are also dependant on the ethos of the hospital and its consultant obstetricians. Hospitals' rates of Caesarean section, assisted and normal birth can be found on the 'Dr. Foster' website and also on the 'Birth Choice UK' website.

Problems or concerns can occur during labour and you could be offered a Caesarean section. There are situations when a Caesarean section is absolutely necessary. One reason is when your baby's heart rate drops and remains low for over nine minutes. This is known as a 'foetal bradycardia'. In most instances his heart rate should recover before six minutes and this is most common after an epidural and their extra doses or 'top ups'. Your baby's heart rate will occasionally drop for up to three minutes and this is commonly a sign that his cord a being compressed. Any longer than this and your midwife will summon assistance and at the same time she will move you onto your left side and lay you flat. This removes the weight of your baby from your large vessels and increases blood flow to your uterus. These steps along with giving you fluid through a small plastic tube or 'cannula' in your hand are usually all that is required to rectify this.

It is extremely rare for your baby's heart rate to remain low for up to nine minutes. If your baby's heart rate was normal before then it is highly likely he is simply taking slightly longer than average time to raise his heart rate again. However, if he was showing signs of distress prior to the drop in heart rate he probably needs to be born immediately. During these nine minutes more people will enter your room to discuss the best course of action. Your midwife will keep you informed of the developing situation and as baby's bradycardia (slow heart beat) approaches nine minutes an anaesthetist will become involved.

At the nine minute mark the decision will be taken to perform a category I emergency Caesarean section. If you have an epidural your anaesthetist may give you medication so it is effective for surgery however, in some circumstances a general anaesthetic is necessary.

Everything moves quickly from here and it can be a frightening experience, although the atmosphere in the room is usually very calm with each member of medical staff playing a role. You will need to give written or verbal consent to the Caesarean section. Saying 'yes' suffices for verbal consent and moving from your bed to the operating table is known as 'implied' consent.

Anaesthetists on labour wards, in certain circumstances are able to perform a regional spinal anaesthetic quicker than a general anaesthetic. The method of anaesthesia however will be their decision and they will tend to opt for the quickest and safest method. You may prefer to have a general anaesthetic, usually due to fear and panic. These are higher risk, do not offer the same post-operative pain relief and you are unaware of the birth. Regardless of everything going on around you, your baby should be able to cope with his heart rate being low or 'bradycardic' for around 20 minutes; enough time to arrange for the birth.

In theatre

Theatres are busy with medical staff, but they all have necessary jobs to do. Firstly, a needle will be placed in your hand if it has not already been fitted earlier. During this time there is a chance that your baby's heart rate will have risen and returned to normal by this point. If this is the case staff will monitor him for a period of time and if there are no concerns they may perform a foetal blood sample. If this result is normal then you may be returned to your room to continue with your labour.

If a general anaesthetic is required your partner will be asked to leave theatre but if you are having a spinal or epidural anaesthetic he can stay to offer support. Your spinal will be sited with you in a sitting position and once sited you will then be assisted to lie flat and moved onto a tilt. A midwife will then pass a catheter into your bladder at the same time as the obstetricians begin to prepare your skin with lotion. You will hear lots of chatter between members of the team as Caesarean section instruments are counted and checked.

In an emergency such as this it will have taken 10 minutes to get to this point.

Once the Caesarean section begins your baby will normally be born in less than one minute. A small incision will have been made at your bikini line and once he is born your placenta will then be removed through the same incision. Your baby will probably need assistance to breathe when he is born and therefore he will be taken immediately to the paediatricians in theatre to be assessed and resuscitated if necessary.

Your midwife remains with you to keep you updated and offer support and you should both direct all questions to her. Depending on how your baby has coped he may be passed to you for skin to skin contact or taken to the neonatal unit for observation and treatment.

Other situations that require a 'Category I' emergency Caesarean section will be if a foetal blood sample result pH is lower than 7.20, however, the closer the result to this figure the less the rush to the operating theatre. However they will still aim to deliver your baby within 30 minutes of this result. If the test shows a pH much lower than 7.20 then result of this test is much lower than the pH 7.20 cut off then it may be necessary to deliver your baby in a shorter time.

More common reasons for C-sections are when there are concerns over your baby's heart rate and medical staff are unable to perform a foetal blood sample to confirm that he is not distressed. It may also be the case that you yourself are causing your midwife and obstetrician concern, for example if you are progressing slowly or have extremely high blood pressure. In these instances you would undergo, what is known as a 'Category II' emergency Caesarean section, and NICE recommends that your baby is born within 45 minutes. This extra time enables you to calmly go through the consent form and ask necessary questions. You may even wish to question whether a Caesarean section is necessary.

If you are booked for an elective Caesarean section and you attend labour ward in labour before that date you will be counselled about whether you wish a vaginal birth.

It may be the case that you have attended labour ward in very early labour and are found to have a breech presentation and are booked for elective Caesarean section. If you fall into this category and have recently eaten and your labour is unlikely to fully establish within six hours then your contraction will be delayed by that time. This reduces the risk of inhaling vomit under general anaesthetic and you could be added to the elective Caesarean list the following day.

Regardless of the category of Caesarean section the process is exactly the same albeit at a different pace.

Following the Birth

Your baby will be assessed immediately after his Caesarean birth and given to you for skin to skin contact if nothing is amiss. The entire operation usually takes around 30 minutes. It may be shorter depending on the amount of Caesarean sections you have had before and the experience of your obstetrician. After surgery the theatre team will roll you onto your bed and any soiled areas will be cleaned and dried. Your baby will then be placed in bed with you and you will both be transferred to a recovery area for observation.

Recovery

You will be observed for signs of bleeding or reaction to the anaesthetic in the recovery area. Your baby will also be assessed and within one hour of his birth your midwife or recovery nurse will help you to breastfeed. If you have had a general anaesthetic and wish to breastfeed you can ask your midwife beforehand to help you with this if you are still asleep. She will have to touch your breast in order to do this so will need your consent however the initial breastfeed within that time is very important.

Postnatal Wards

Once time on the recovery ward has established all is well with you and baby you'll both be transferred to the postnatal ward. You will have a catheter fitted to ensure your bladder is emptying whilst you have no sensation to pass urine. You will stay in hospital an average of two to three days after a Caesarean birth, but this does vary.

On the postnatal ward you will be encouraged to mobilise as soon as possible, usually around six hours or the following morning. Being quickly out of bed helps reduce risks of blood clots, which are increased with any surgery and to further reduce the risk of blood clots you will be provided with compression stockings and blood thinning drugs for seven days. Your recovery will take longer than that of a vaginal birth and it is important to follow the advice of your midwife and obstetrician. Many women will do too much too soon and find that they bleed more heavily and have more pain, so take it easy.

Pathway to Caesarean Section

1. Concerns about you or your baby have been identified.
2. Explanations given as to why you need a Caesarean section.
3. Consent for the operation discussed and obtained.
4. Anaesthetist is now present to talk to you about your options for anaesthesia.
5. Move into the operating theatre.
6. Have your anaesthetic (and cannula if needed).
7. Catheter inserted into your bladder.
8. Paediatricians will now be present in theatre.
9. Baby will be born and given to you or assessed by the paediatricians.
10. If your baby is well and you wish he will be weighed and checked over.
11. Once the surgery is over you will be transferred to a recovery area.
12. Once you are suitably recovered you will be transferred to a postnatal ward or room.

Chapter 16

Emergencies

Expectant women are assessed at either high or low risk of developing problems. Although many of these complications are rare it is right to mention them in this book, but please do not worry because there is little chance of them affecting your pregnancy.

Women and their partners can suffer psychologically when emergency situations occur because they are unaware of what is happening. There is little time to explain the situation and offer support until it is over.

The word *emergency* conjures up feelings of dread in us all. We may think of television programmes but what we rarely do is place ourselves in that position. Luckily only a very small number of us will find ourselves there and the vital factor for everyone is that everything that can be done is done. Your birth partner should calmly keep you informed of what is happening and if possible why, and the staff, though busy, should be able to keep telling him what is happening. Your birth partner is not legally able to give consent on your behalf, so it's best to keep calm and listen.

Shoulder Dystocia

Shoulder dystocia effects one in every two hundred babies. When your baby's head is born his shoulders should come down onto your pelvic floor and turn ninety degrees in order to come out. For some babies the shoulder sitting under the top of your pelvis, your 'pubis' becomes wedged just above it preventing your baby from being born. When this happens your midwife will pull the emergency buzzer in your room or in a homebirth she will call an ambulance.

If you are on the bed, while she is waiting for help she will lower the back of your bed and remove any pillows that may be there. When help arrives staff will push your knees together and towards your ears. This is known as 'McRoberts' position and up to 90 percent of babies will be born using this position. In this position you will be encouraged to keep pushing. After a set amount of time, usually 30 seconds, another member of staff will press on your lower abdomen just above your pelvis.

This technique pushes your baby's shoulder into a different position making the diameter smaller and helping him to be born. Again this is undertaken for a set amount of time, usually 30-60 seconds. During this procedure another member of staff will remove the end of your bed and the paediatricians will have been summoned.

If pressing on your pelvis is unsuccessful then a member of the team will then insert their hand into your vagina. They will try to manually turn your baby round or deliver his bottom arm using various techniques. If this too is unsuccessful and if you can move, you will be assisted onto all fours and the techniques then repeated. Whilst stuck he may not be receiving sufficient amounts of oxygen so the manoeuvres are done quickly and efficiently. It may take several minutes for your baby to be born and it is likely he will not be breathing when he is. The paediatricians will be present in your room for his birth and he will be immediately taken to them for assessment and any necessary resuscitation.

After his assessment and possible treatment, if he is well enough he will be handed to you for skin to skin. If he needs to be monitored on the neonatal unit then you will be able to visit him as soon as your placenta has been removed and any tears repaired.

Because this emergency is usually over quickly most team members will have a vital job and there may not be someone available to explain all that is happening. The team will remain calm and in control and talking is usually kept to a minimum so that vital information is not missed and team members can concentrate.

Once you are sufficiently recovered your midwife and obstetrician will debrief you on the events and you will be encouraged to ask any questions you wish. One of these questions may be '*Why did this happen*?', or '*Why didn't you predict this?*' The most frustrating part of shoulder dystocia is its unpredictability. There are warning signs that a problem may be imminent but not until the head is being born. It affects big and small babies alike. If you are having a big baby your pelvis will normally be a suitable size for a straightforward labour.

Performing an elective Caesarean section when a large baby is anticipated would be unnecessary and subject you to unnecessary risk. A history of shoulder dystocia puts you at higher risk of another and because of this if you have a subsequent pregnancy you will be referred to a consultant obstetrician and the option of Caesarean section will be discussed with you.

If you feel that you are suffering from anxiety it may be that you need to discuss this with your midwife, consultant or G.P. who will be able to arrange some counselling.

Cord Prolapse

This occurs when your baby's cord slips in front of his head after his waters have broken and the pressure of his head on the cord will cause an erratic heart rate pattern or a sustained drop in his heart rate. The incidence of this is 1 to 6 women in 1,000, however with breech presentation it is slightly higher at 1 woman in 100. If his cord does prolapse it will be picked up on his heart rate trace or as your midwife listens to his heart rate after your waters have broken. If there are concerns you may have suffered from a cord prolapse then your midwife or obstetrician will perform a vaginal examination to check. If this confirms a cord prolapse then she will ask you partner to pull the emergency buzzer in your room.

She will then ask you to quickly move onto all fours with your head resting against your bed or the floor and with your bottom in the air. She will then gently push your baby's head upwards to relieve pressure on his cord. She will be unable to remove her fingers from your vagina so if you have an epidural she will ask your partner to assist you to move onto your left side.

By this time help should have arrived in your room and an assessment will quickly be made of the situation. If your cervix is fully dilated and his head is low then your midwife or obstetrician may opt for you to push him out or failing that perform an assisted birth.

If your cervix is not fully dilated or his head is high then you will be asked to consent to a Caesarean section. The speed at which this needs to be done will depend on a number of factors:

If your midwife's attempts to raise your baby's head with her fingers fails to work, you will be immediately moved to theatre for a Category I Caesarean section. On the transfer to theatre your midwife will need to keep her fingers in your vagina and you will remain on all fours. This is a most undignified position although you will be fully covered with a sheet and the corridors on labour ward will be cleared of visitors. There will be little time to spare and you will probably require a general anaesthetic as your position will make a spinal extremely difficult and time consuming for your anaesthetist.

As soon as possible your midwife will inform your partner of the birth and keep him up to date with the surgery. If the manoeuvre that your midwife is using to push your baby's head off his cord is relieving his erratic heart rate then a catheter will be passed into your bladder. It will be filled with fluid, and as your bladder fills it will lift your uterus and your baby's head from the cord.

If this continues to relieve the pressure as effectively as your midwife's fingers then she will be able to remove them from your vagina. This should allow more time to perform a Caesarean section. This may also allow the anaesthetist to perform a spinal anaesthetic although it is more likely that a general anaesthetic will be performed.

Once in the recovery area you will be updated as to what has happened. If your baby has needed to be transferred to the neonatal unit you will be able to visit him as soon as you are more awake. If he has remained with you your midwife or recovery nurse will assist you to breastfeed and your recovery will be as any other Caesarean section.

Postpartum Haemorrhage

This is a loss of blood following birth of greater than 500 millilitres in 24 hours, however most women are able to tolerate a blood loss of up to one litre before they begin to feel unwell.

Blood loss is notoriously difficult to estimate and because of this the incidence of postpartum haemorrhage is noted to be anything from five to 25 percent. Some studies examining the average amount of blood loss for vaginal births and Caesarean section found it to be 400-600 millilitres and 1 litre respectively.

The point at which women will become unwell varies enormously and is dependent on their size, weight and the level of iron in their blood before birth however women rarely bleed so heavily that they become extremely unwell.

Some 35 women in 10,000 births lose more than 2½ litres and any heavy blood loss is managed quickly and efficiently in order to minimise that risk. If you do begin to bleed heavily it may happen immediately following the birth or later when you are on the postnatal ward.

The four causes of postpartum haemorrhage:

- It may be that your uterus does not contract   strongly enough to constrict the blood flow and will require drugs to help with this. This is the most common cause of blood loss and your midwife will immediately massage your uterus in an attempt to stimulate a contraction
- You may also have small parts of your placenta or blood clots in your uterus which will also prevent it from contracting effectively. They will need to be removed in order to resolve this problem
- There may be lacerations to your birth canal that are bleeding heavily and will require repair to stop this blood loss. This can be caused by your body lacking or not producing enough clotting factors.
- This is the rarest cause and any problems with your blood's ability to clot will be identified antenatally and a plan for management put in place. Specialist drugs and blood products may be needed.

When postpartum haemorrhaging occurs help will be summoned by pressing the emergency buzzer and your midwife will begin massaging your uterus in an effort to make it contract. While she is doing this other members of the labour ward team will have arrived.

Everything needs to be done quickly so there will be little time to explain fully what is happening. A member of the team will place one or two cannulas in your hand and draw some blood to test your iron levels and clotting. Your blood group will also be checked in case a blood transfusion is needed.

Your blood pressure, pulse and oxygen saturations will be taken regularly and you will be given intravenous fluid. If your uterus is relaxing you will be medicated through a vein, which may cause you to vomit. Another member of the team, usually an obstetrician, will examine your perineum to see whether or not the blood loss is in relation to a tear. Your uterus will also be checked for clots. Once complete a catheter will then be used to empty your bladder.

In most cases the drugs used or repairs to a tear are sufficient to control bleeding. Your placenta is checked to ensure it is complete as any tissue remaining in your uterus may stop it from contracting efficiently.

In rare cases bleeding can be caused by your blood not clotting effectively. This is treated with specialist drugs and management. If these drugs fail to stop the bleeding, your uterus continues to relax, or there is tissue in your uterus preventing it from contracting, then you will be moved to theatre to ensure adequate lighting and pain relief while you undergo examination and treatment, usually under general anaesthetic. Your partner and your baby will remain in your room while you are transferred to theatre.

Following the procedure you will be returned to the labour ward for observation of your blood pressure, pulse and other vital signs, and for close observation of any further blood loss. Blood tests will then be repeated to check iron levels and if they are very low you will be counselled about receiving a blood transfusion. It is also important that your partner is also present at debrief to allay his worries.

At home take it easy for a few weeks and it may take months before you feel back to normal and your blood supply is replenished. Ensure you have help around the house and for the first few weeks concentrate on nothing other than feeding your baby.

Chapter 17

Giving Birth

Giving Birth with an Epidural

If you have an epidural and cannot feel the pressure of your baby's head, your midwife will be reminding you of where and when to push. She will encourage you to push as if you were opening your bowels. You may become frustrated as you may feel you are not making progress, but your birth partner and midwife will encourage you to carry on.

With an epidural it is important you do not resort to closed glottis pushing, or the 'Valsalva Manoeuvre', when you take a deep breath, hold it and push down into your bottom. The problem with this technique is it increases the pressure in your chest and causes a reduction in the blood flow to your uterus and therefore your baby. To avoid this place your fist in your mouth and make a seal with your lips. Ensuring that no air escapes, you will now push with the contractions. This technique avoids the potential problems associated with the 'Valsalva Manoeuvre' and ensures that you are able to focus your pushing in the right area.

With an epidural you should expect to push for at least an hour and sometimes two. Some labour wards apply time limits to this stage of labour, but they are arbitrary. The usual time limits for the second stage in hospital guidelines are four hours from the time your cervix was fully dilated. Standard guidelines suggest offering an assisted birth if there has been no descent or rotation of your baby's head after pushing for one hour. If there has been descent and progress most midwives and obstetricians will offer you an assisted birth after two hours of pushing, unless your baby's birth is imminent. If your baby is still back to back you may need one hour simply to turn him round to the correct position. When you push with a baby in a back to back position you have to push him into your pelvis in an unnatural way. If you have an epidural your pelvic floor is more lax so he has even further to descend into your pelvis before he reaches your pelvic floor. Only when his head presses against your pelvic floor does he have the resistance needed to allow his head to turn. The slope of your pelvic floor, as his head meets it, directs it forward and causes him to turn.

If after one hour your baby's head has not descended then ask if he has turned. If he has then there has been progress. If there are no concerns about him or you then it is safe to carry on pushing. The hard work has been done and you may only need another 30 to 40 minutes of pushing before your baby is born. There are some facts you need to be aware of. The length of your labour correlates to the amount of blood you lose at the birth. The longer you are in labour the more blood you tend to lose.

Also, when pushing, the pudendal nerve, which supplies the bladder, may be stretched. This can cause you to have difficulty passing urine after the birth so you may be offered a catheter for 24 hours to rest it.

Assisted Birth

Sometimes, despite everything that you have done to avoid one, and it is usually dependent on the shape of your pelvis, it is necessary to perform an assisted birth. Your baby could be showing signs of distress and it may be safer for you and him to have an assisted birth. Your baby's head will probably be too low in your pelvis to make a Caesarean section a safe option. Also, a Caesarean section at full dilatation of your cervix carries a higher risk of infection and bleeding at this stage of your labour.

Forceps or ventouse is a decision taken by the midwife or obstetrician carrying out the procedure. A forceps birth is usually carried out when your baby's head is still not visible when you push or there is a lot of swelling on the top of his head. If your baby has become distressed and needs to be born straightaway, your midwife or obstetrician will normally opt for a forceps birth as it is most likely to be successful and quicker than a ventouse.

Babies delivered by forceps can receive marks or bruises to the skin on the face and occasionally grazes where the forceps were applied, while babies delivered by ventouse may suffer headaches caused by a 'chignon' or swelling of their head.

A ventouse birth is no riskier for you than a normal birth, however a forceps birth will increase your risk of third degree tears and you will need an episiotomy. If a ventouse birth is attempted when your baby's head is high the suction cup will usually displace and need to be reapplied. If this happens a few times your midwife or obstetrician will revert to forceps. Likewise if there is a lot of swelling on your baby's head then they will be unable to apply the ventouse and forceps will need to be applied.

Forceps Birth

If you've had no pain relief you will be offered a spinal anaesthetic or a pudendal block. Both offer excellent pain relief with benefits and drawbacks. A Spinal anaesthetic requires you to give birth in theatre with an anaesthetist present. You will be numb from the waist down - this type of anaesthetic is used for Caesarean section so you will be in bed for at least six hours.

A pudendal block works in the same way as an anaesthetic you would be given by your dentist. It 'blocks' the nerve pathways to the lower part of your pelvis. You should feel no pain but you will feel pulling and pushing. The benefits of a pudendal block are you can give birth in your labour ward room and you can walk immediately afterwards.

In both cases the delivery is the same. Firstly, your legs are placed into lithotomy poles attached to the side of your bed. Your perineal area is cleaned and draped with sterile towels and a catheter is passed to drain your bladder then removed. Another vaginal examination is performed to confirm the position of your baby is in before forceps are applied one at a time. When the forceps are in place your midwife will either feel for contractions or encourage you to push when you have one. As you push your midwife or obstetrician will gently guide your baby's head out and perform an episiotomy, a cut to the skin and muscle of the area between your vagina and anus, just before his head is born. The forceps are then removed and with your next contraction they will help you to deliver the rest of your baby. If needed your baby will be taken the resuscitation table and be assessed by a paediatrician, midwife or nurse, but it is more common for him to be placed on your stomach after he is born and to be assessed there. Following this your placenta will be delivered and your perineum sutured but it is unlikely that you'll be aware of this as you welcome your baby into your family.

Ventouse Birth

The cup of the ventouse that sits on your baby's head is about the size of a tennis ball which has been cut in half and is smaller than his head. Because of this there is no need for pain relief unless you request some. You will be helped into lithotomy position and, as with a forceps birth your perineum will be cleaned and draped with sterile towels and your bladder emptied with a catheter. As you push, your midwife or obstetrician will gently guide your baby's head out and once his head is born, remove the ventouse cup. Usually, there is no need to perform an episiotomy and baby is usually placed straight onto your stomach. As with forceps deliveries, if needed, he will be taken to the resuscitation table to be assessed. Once you have your baby in your arms your placenta will then be delivered and any tears repaired.

For some women there will be disappointment that they required a forceps or ventouse birth especially when they followed all the advice given to them. This should not be viewed as some sort of failure but a testament to your strength and endurance that you managed to give birth after such a difficult labour. You should tell yourself 'I worked hard for that forceps birth' and mean it.

If you used an epidural for pain relief recognise that it was the only option and you could well have required an assisted labour anyway. Labour and birth is a means to an end. We can strive to enjoy its amazing journey, but ultimately the way we give birth is predestined by the shape of our pelvis and the size of our babies.

Vaginal Breech Birth

INCIDENCE

Most babies at term will be head down, but some will decide that they are more comfortable bottom first or 'breech'. As pregnancies progress the incidence of breech presentations lessens and this is why premature babies are at a higher risk of breech presentation. There are three types of breech presentation:

- Breech with straight legs towards his head (frank or extended) – the most common and found in 85 percent of cases.
- Breech with flexed legs (complete) – in a cross-legged or kneeling position.
- Footling (incomplete) with one or both legs extended downwards towards your cervix.

Most babies with a breech presentation are delivered by Caesarean section. Your community midwife will ask for a presentation scan if there is a suspicion your baby is in a breech position. If you baby has been identified as being a breech presentation you will be offered an 'external cephalic version' before labour. In around half of those undertaken your baby will turn to head down. If the external cephalic version was unsuccessful you will be counselled by your obstetrician about whether you want a Caesarean section or a vaginal breech birth. If labour begins and he is still in a breech position you will be offered a vaginal birth or Caesarean section.

Reasons for a Breech Presentation

Reasons for babies to be in a breech presentation include:

- A lax uterus usually associated with the number of pregnancies you have had.
- Uterine anomalies (e.g. bicornuate or septate uterus).
- Placenta praevia – where your placenta covers your cervix.
- An abnormal pelvis.
- Maternal smoking.
- Babies with hydrocephalus (water on the brain)
- Multiple pregnancies, such as twins.
- Excess fluid known as polyhydramnios.
- Reduced fluid known as oligohydramnios.
- A low birth weight baby.
- A premature baby.
- A previous breech baby

Giving Birth to a Breech Baby

In the case of a breech birth labour the obstetrician will normally catch your baby, rather than your midwife. If a midwife does catch your baby she will be very experienced in vaginal breech birth.

If you are in labour then there are some differences to note and it is usual that an obstetrician will help you give birth rather than your midwife. This ensures that they gain the necessary experience and they may also feel it appropriate to support another more junior obstetrician or your midwife to assist you to give birth. This is also important as it allows junior, inexperienced staff to gain these skills and enable them to offer more vaginal breech births to more women. Midwives also need to be proficient in vaginal breech birth as there are occasions during homebirths and busy periods on labour ward where obstetricians may not immediately available.

Your baby's breech presentation may not be discovered until you arrive at hospital in advanced labour. If your baby's bottom is already visible at your vagina then a Caesarean section may not be the safest option for either of you.

Your baby's heart rate will be monitored continuously and any concerns will be acted upon, however, all other aspects of your assisted labour should be no different from that of a baby coming head first. Forceps and an episiotomy might be needed to guide your baby's head out as slowly as possible or a standing or squatting position might be suggested to aid the manoeuvres your baby need to make to be born.

In hospital you will probably be on a bed with your legs in lithotomy position. However, this position is not necessary until your baby's bottom has become visible. In that situation the foot of your bed will be removed to allow your baby to hang down as he is born.

Because junior doctors and inexperienced midwives have to learn, you may be asked whether you mind more people in the room to observe a breech birth. A paediatrician, obstetrician, your midwife and partner will be present. If that is all you want, just say.

Babies will pop out by themselves so midwives abide by the '*hands off the breech*' rule. You will be encouraged to push with your contractions and your baby's bottom will slowly emerge. His legs will appear and if they don't come out then the practitioner will gently flick them out. As baby is pushed further down your pelvis help may be needed to free his arms.

After his body is born it will be covered with a swab to keep him warm. The weight of his body, on your next contraction, is usually sufficient for his head to be born.

Most breech babies are purple or blue when born and tend not to be breathing. All they need is the stimulation of the cold air and rubbing with a towel to begin breathing. If this is insufficient he will be taken to the paediatrician to help with his breathing, then given back to you for skin to skin contact.

Twins

Today, with ultrasound scans and routine antenatal appointments, unidentified twin pregnancies are virtually unheard of in the United Kingdom. With assisted conception and IVF pregnancies twins are increasingly common. There are two types of twin pregnancies; these are dizygotic, where two eggs have been fertilised and monozygotic, one egg is fertilised and divides into two.

Dizygotic twins are non-identical, have two placentas and these pregnancies are the least complicated of the two but are still considered high risk. Monozygotic twins are called identical and are higher risk because of a shared placenta and possible cord entanglement. Although approximately 50 percent of twins are delivered by Caesarean section, that still leaves another 50 percent born vaginally.

For vaginal birth of twins it is advised that labour is induced before 38 weeks of pregnancy as the average gestation for a twin pregnancy is around 37 weeks. This is because as with any post term pregnancy the risk of stillbirth increases after 38 weeks and if your twins' labour does not begin before 37 weeks you will usually be offered a date for induction.

As with any induction of labour it can take a few days to ripen your cervix enough to be able to induce labour. Also, caring for a lady with a twin pregnancy in labour is more complicated than a single pregnancy and therefore induction of labour has more chance of being delayed because more medical staff will be required.

Care in Labour

Whether your labour is induced or spontaneous your care in labour does not differ. Whilst on the labour ward both babies will be monitored on a continuous heart rate trace. A thin plastic tube or 'cannula' is placed in your hand for intravenous fluids. You may also be offered an epidural, however, there are disadvantages to using an epidural for pain relief namely that it increases your risk of an assisted delivery.

Giving Birth to Twins

With a twin pregnancy your first baby tends to cause few problems and his labour and birth should progress as any other. As he is born your midwife will ask for another member of the team to be present. Hospitals have different guidelines on who should be present. There might be two midwives, an obstetrician and two paediatricians, or there may only be two midwives. Some midwives and obstetricians prefer to stabilise your second baby in place as your first baby is born to prevent him moving into an unsafe position although there is no strong evidence to support this practice either way.

Once your first baby is born he will be placed on your stomach and, if he is crying and there are no concerns, he will remain there until his cord is clamped and cut.

Because you have to give birth to a second baby you can ask your partner to give your first baby skin to skin contact. This is now common practice on most labour wards, and blankets are provided to protect dad's modesty.

With your baby now with dad your midwife or obstetrician will perform a palpation of your abdomen to assess whether the second twin's head or bottom have descended into your pelvis. This may take a few minutes and during that time it may be necessary to commence the hormone drip.

When your second baby's head or bottom is felt to be in your pelvis your midwife or obstetrician will carry out another vaginal examination to determine whether or not they can break your waters. Once your waters have been broken they will wait until you begin to feel the need to push again and your second baby will be born; this time for you to have skin to skin contact.

Occasionally, second twins move into positions where a vaginal birth is deemed too dangerous and at that time you will be consented for a category one Caesarean section. The anaesthetist will determine what type of anaesthesia you have and whether or not your partner will be able to accompany you to the operation theatre. If your baby is felt to be in danger but can be born vaginally then it may be necessary for your obstetrician to perform either a breech extraction or a forceps birth. Either of these situations will be worrying but your midwife will keep you informed at all times and be assured that you will have the most experienced team on labour ward caring for you all.

After both babies are born your placenta will be delivered. This placenta will be twice the size of a normal placenta and your uterus will have been stretched further than in a single pregnancy. For these reasons you are at greater risk of a haemorrhage and your midwife and obstetrician will monitor your blood loss closely and will wish to manage your third stage of labour with drugs.

If you have given birth vaginally and your babies were born after 37 weeks' gestation then, providing there are no other concerns, you will be able to go home as soon as you feel ready. Twins, however, do take some getting used to and perhaps a few nights stay on a postnatal ward will help with that adjustment, especially if you are breastfeeding.

For just under 50 percent of women at least one of their twins will spend time in the neonatal unit. This is primarily due to them being underweight and earlier than 37 weeks'. If you are expecting twins, or any multiple pregnancy, it is a good idea for both of you to sleep with your babies' blankets to transmit your scent onto them. If they are admitted to the neonatal unit you can ask the staff to place them on these blankets ensuring they can smell you at all times.

Water birth

"Pure water is the world's first and foremost medicine"
Slovakian Proverb

Water birth is not a new phenomenon or trendy fad. There are tales of South Pacific Islanders giving birth in rock pools and Egyptian Pharaohs being born in lakes.

Some obstetricians in the mid-1980s, most notably French, believed birth had become unnecessarily medicalised to the benefit of the doctors and detriment of the women and their babies. They thought the transition from the womb through a quick and mechanically forced labour into a cold, noisy, bright environment traumatised infants for life.

The peaceful transition from the warm water of their mother's womb to the warm water of the birthing pool seemed less traumatic and women benefited as they were calmer, more relaxed and less reliant on strong forms of pain relief. Water birth babies were noted to be calmer, more settled and because of the lack of pain relief, less likely to display feeding problems.

Little research had been done on the subject of water birth and the medical fraternity was distrustful that something so natural and simple could be used as an alternative to drugs and instruments. Midwives too struggled to champion this method but over time water births have proved very popular.

Safety

In your uterus baby does not breathe. His lungs are filled with fluid and your placenta provides him with oxygen and removes waste products. Babies gasp when they are born due to a negative pressure in their chest sucking air into the lungs. This air will displace fluid water in his lungs and after a few breaths his lungs are clear. A number of stimuli cause a baby to gasp at birth; exposure to cold is usually the first reason, and when the umbilical cord is cut the build-up of carbon dioxide and low oxygen will also trigger a gasp.

Fears that the 'dive reflex'- the reflex used by all mammals in order to submerge and dive in water – will kick in are unfounded. This reflex is triggered by water no warmer than 21 degrees Celsius. The diving reflex will not be triggered in a birthing pool which is just below normal body temperature. It is the lack of the usual stimuli to take a breath that will prevent the initiation of breathing.

Benefits

The benefits of using water for labour and birth are numerous. The warm water helps to relax your muscles and the buoyancy of the water helps lessen the work for your muscles. Your body can then divert that unused energy, in the form of glucose, to the muscles of your uterus, where they are at their greatest need. In water you can change position more easily and frequently and the relaxation encourages the production of oxytocin and endorphins, helping labour to progress with natural pain relief.

A study found women who opted for water birth were half as likely to use pain relief compared to those who did not although you are still free to use gas and air and your partner can still rub your back in water.

Also, there is no extra risk of tears to your perineum during a water birth and it is thought the pressure of the water against your perineum gives it support. If you do suffer a tear which needs repairing then your water-logged tissue will have to return to normal before this can be done, usually after around an hour following your water birth.

One drawback of a water birth is the lack of closeness with your partner, but providing the hospital allows it, there is no reason why he shouldn't be able to join you in the pool.

In relation to clothing, some women prefer to be naked while others will wear bikinis, underwear or a nightdress in the water. A word of warning though, should you open your bowels in the water and depending on your hospitals policies, he may be expected to scoop it out. The faeces itself is not a danger to your baby as its diluted but you should avoid letting it get into your eyes or open wounds.

There are few ways to give birth as beneficial as immersion in water. Each labour ward or birthing centre will have set criteria for water birth and most will accept women with otherwise straightforward labours who require a heart rate trace as an underwater monitoring unit can be used for this.

Do bear in mind that the birthing pool may be in use so when you arrive in labour inform your midwife of your wishes immediately. Additionally, although water is an effective form of pain relief, it can slow the birthing process if used in the latent or early phase of labour. In active labour, providing your cervix has opened to around five centimetres, this should not be a factor.

There may be occasions when your midwife will advise you to leave the pool and they may include:

- If your baby's head is exposed to the air, no matter how small a part of it
- If your contractions have slowed down
- If your pulse has increased
- If your baby's heart rate has changed
- If your baby has passed meconium
- If you begin to bleed
- If your temperature begins to rise
- If you need to pass urine and your midwife wishes to measure it
- For vaginal examinations

In a normal healthy pregnancy with no risk factors the use water for labour and birth should be the first thing you use for pain relief. Even if the thought of giving birth in the water frightens or even repulses you please try it, you will be amazed at its effect.

Transition and Pushing

Transition is a phase of labour that it will affect almost every woman. It is the final phase of your birth journey - pushing. Transition lasts around 20 minutes, during which time your behaviour may become completely out of character and you may notice an overwhelming anxiety. You may panic and will most likely frighten the life out of your partner, but this is normal and not to be feared.

Transition is common and your midwife and partner should support you through it with reassurance. Transition is intense, not because the pain is worse, but because of the sensation that you are no longer in control. This is true; transition is the precursor to the second stage of your labour, the pushing stage, and is in some way preparing you for imminent motherhood. Now is the time many women, if they have avoided strong pain relief earlier, will request them and almost every woman will utter the immortal words *"I cannot do it!"* The answer that your birth partner and midwife will give is *"You can do it and you are"*. This is true; you have come to the final part of birth and are almost at the end of this journey; in a few minutes the feeling of anxiety will go.

Your partner may notice you start to shake and shiver and may ask if you're cold. If he asks that question the birth of your baby is not far away. You partner may feel that you need pain relief - it is important he keeps this to himself. Now is not the time to reinforce negative thoughts. Your midwife knows once this phase has passed you will be ready to push. She will encourage you through this phase and help you to manage your emotions. You may feel she is not listening to you, especially if you have requested pain relief. They will tell you it will not last for much longer. They may be firm to help your breathing exercises but they will not touch you because you will not want that. You will shout, maybe cry, and it is important that your birth partner recognises this is not caused by pain but by primal instinct. Reassurance is what you need. You may be requesting an epidural but what you really want is for someone to tell you that this is normal and will be over soon. Do not fight it, embrace it. Try to visualise the end and that your body is gently positioning your baby ready for his birth.

Foreknowledge of the transition stage and its effects means it should not hold the same fear. It may actually pass you by and only later will your partner tell you that you did act out of character.

Transition is followed by a serene calmness and you will feel as if your labour has stopped. The contractions that overcame you a moment since are barely present now. This is the time to relax, to take deep breaths and prepare yourself for the next stage. The next contraction you feel will probably make you want to push and that means your baby wants to be born. During this stage you will feel immense relief and a calm sensation of wellbeing. This is the effect of oxytocin as your baby's head descends through your pelvis and onto your pelvic floor. On this journey your body is preparing him for the final stage and allows him a brief rest. This calm stage lasts for about 15-20 minutes and for some women they will have no contractions during that time. This will give you the perfect opportunity to rest and possibly empty your bladder.

When your contractions start again they will feel very different. They will become purposeful and you will not feel the same intensity in your abdomen. You will first have the sensation that you need to open your bowels and it will be a strong sensation. You will feel the only way to get comfortable is to push but you will still have the ability to stop yourself. This is known as feeling 'rectal pressure'. Following this your body will begin to make you push and you will probably be unaware that you are. Your midwife however will recognise this stage and may even ask you if you need to push. *Needing* to push is very different from *wanting* to push. By wanting to push you have control over it but when you need to push you no longer have that control.

Initially it will be at the height of your contractions and that sensation will increase over time. Your baby's head will now be pressing down on your pelvic floor and distending the muscles surrounding your vagina. This will initiate the 'Ferguson Reflex' which will produce another surge of oxytocin and increase the force of your contractions. The sensation is not painful but felt as an overwhelming urge to push. By this point your cervix will be fully dilated, none will be felt in front of your baby's head and you will be in the second stage of labour. It will not be necessary for your midwife to confirm this by carrying out a vaginal examination but you may want her to. It will be an academic point though, if you are unable to stop yourself from pushing, discovering that your cervix is open 9cm will not change that.

There is no evidence that pushing when your cervix is open 8cm or more will cause problems with your labour or damage your cervix. At this point you will lose the ability to stop yourself from pushing and will be making low guttural noises as the contractions make you push. Give in to it and push. Trust your body and don't be afraid, there will be no pain, just a feeling of release and empowerment.

Positions for Birth

You have now spent some time in the second stage of labour. Your baby has moved down through your pelvis and the top of his head can be seen at the height of your contractions. You will probably find that the guttural noises you have been making become louder and you may not be aware of this. Your midwife will now be preparing for the imminent birth of your baby.

Upright Positions

You should be encouraged to make noise at this point, it is a natural response. You may find, if you are standing, that your knees will bend with each push as you bear down. If you are on all fours you will find that you move your bottom towards the floor and as it subsides you rock forwards again. Using both of these positions will enable you to face your partner and listen to his words of encouragement. You will also be able to look into his eyes and focus on your birth. If you have decided that lying down is the position you wish to give birth in then try being on your left side as it has been shown to reduce tears to your perineum and allows your coccyx to move out of the way of your baby's head

Birthing Stool

Of all the positions for giving birth this is the one where your partner is most involved. Sit on the birthing stool with your partner sitting behind and he can cocoon you. Your midwife will watch as your baby's head begins to stretch the skin of your perineum. Once you stop pushing you will feel him moving back inwards. This is because the bone at the back of his head, his 'occiput', is trying to slip under the front of your pelvis. He will continue to rock backwards and forwards like this, allowing the muscle and skin of your perineum to stretch.

This is the point of labour at which you will instinctively know when to push and when not to. If this is your first baby the skin has never been stretched before and it will take a while until your baby is ready to be born. If this is your second or third baby then you may be asked by your midwife to breath or 'pant' straightaway. As your baby's head crowns you will scream, this is known as the 'Primal Scream' and it is not in a response to pain it is, as the name suggests, primal. When you scream you release all of your energy out of your mouth, with very little directed to your bottom and this allows your baby's head to be breathed out slowly and not forced out.

If you are standing, you will raise yourself up and thrust your hips forward simultaneously, in what is known as the 'Foetal Ejection Reflex'. If you are on the birthing stool you will lift your bottom from the stool and again thrust your hips forwards. Your head will be thrown backwards to rest on your partner's shoulder and at the same time he will witness the birth of his baby. Your baby can then be grasped by you and lifted to your chest. If you give birth in a standing or all fours position then your midwife will catch your baby and pass him to you for skin to skin contact.

Giving Birth in Water

Water births are certainly the gentlest of births. There does not appear to be the same noise and the stages and phases that midwives look for are less apparent. Labour in water is more of a continuum and the birth is merely an extension of that. Depending on your midwife's practice she may or may not use a mirror in the pool and may or may not use gloves. The important thing to remember with a water birth is that it is completely hands off, and for a midwife that is a very humbling experience. You truly see women birthing without any assistance or intervention and they do it with such serenity and calmness. Your midwife will only offer words of encouragement and support and the next thing you will see is your baby floating at the bottom of the pool, his arms outstretched, staring at you. You will, without thinking, reach into the water and gently lift him towards you. He has had such a calm entrance to this world that he is not stressed and only slowly will he feel the cold air that will make him take his first breath. Water babies never cry straightaway. They appear as if they were still in your uterus, nonplussed and relaxed, still waiting to be born.

Following the Birth

You did it! You have brought a brand new life, or lives into this world and with it your lives are changed forever. Your baby, not long ago was placed in your arms and now everyone stares in wonderment at him, gently checking his fingers and toes.

His cord will still be attached, so if your midwife has not already done so, this is usually the time she will discuss the third stage of labour. This stage is the final one and is defined as the stage following the birth of your baby until your placenta and membranes have been delivered. Immediately following your birth you will be moved onto clean pads, any soiled bed linen will be changed and your room will be cleaned and tidied. The only evidence of childbirth will be the baby in your arms and you will be given time with him as a family. You will be encouraged to maintain skin to skin contact for as long as possible and at least until your baby has breastfed as this is known to help initiate his first feed. You will be given as much assistance as you wish to breastfeed and even if you have breastfed before it is wise to ask you midwife for help and advice with his first feed. Even if you are not breastfeeding skin to skin contact has many other benefits and you will be encouraged to do this for as long as possible. During this time your midwife will check your blood pressure, pulse and temperature to ensure that there are no concerns with him or you.

Once you are ready your midwife will weight your baby, put a nappy on him and apply identity bracelets to his ankles. Depending on which hospital you give birth in he may also have a security device attached to him. He will then be checked by your midwife for any obvious problems for which she would need to make a referral to the paediatricians. If this is necessary she will speak to them straightaway and inform you of when or if your baby will be reviewed.

If he does need to have his observations taken then these will be commenced earlier, usually at the time of his birth or close to it. He needn't be moved from skin to skin however, this can all be done with him where he is. At this point you will also be offered a bath or shower and refreshments in the form of tea and toast for you and your birth partners.

Postnatal Bladder Care

Bladder care after birth is just as important as it was during labour. You may have been unable to avoid bruising or stretching your bladder, or the pudendal nerve which supplies sensation to your bladder. If stretching or bruising has occurred you may find it difficult to pass urine or, if you can pass urine, be unable to completely empty your bladder. Over time your bladder may become stretched and inefficient which may later lead to stress incontinence. For this reason your midwife will encourage you to pass urine not long after birth and might measure it. If you cannot pass urine or empty your bladder then she will offer either to scan your bladder or pass a catheter. You could be dehydrated, and scanning your bladder will confirm it is empty; drinking fluids will remedy this.

If a bladder scan shows your bladder contains urine, then your bladder is not functioning properly and you would normally be advised to have a catheter passed into your bladder to rest it for at least 24 hours. After the catheter is removed your bladder will be rescanned after you've passed urine.

If you do require a catheter for an extended period of time it is usual practice to allow you home and return to hospital for its removal and subsequent assessments.

Going Home

You can go home from hospital as early as two to six hours following your birth and so long as you and your baby are healthy most hospitals transfer you both home at that point. This allows enough time to ensure bleeding has settled, you have passed urine with no problems, that your baby has fed and that no problems were identified on his detailed examination. If you are breastfeeding for the first time or are having trouble initiating it then you will be advised to stay on the postnatal ward for specialist assistance.

On leaving hospital you will be given advice leaflets on postnatal care and may be given information to pass to your G.P. and health visitor. If you are a rhesus negative blood group, you may well be given an injection of anti D immunoglobulin.

Hospitals practice differs throughout the country so you would need to confirm this with your midwife.

Part 3

Parenthood

Chapter 18

At Home

Visitors and Visiting

When you arrive home the temptation will be to invite everyone over to meet your new arrival or to visit family members to introduce him. Listen to your body. If it tells you to rest then do so and do not be tempted to run around after visitors no matter how well you feel, that is your partner or other family members' job.

You may find a steady stream of visitors at all times of the day makes it difficult to organise and settle into a feeding pattern with your baby. You will also have been advised to sleep or rest when your baby sleeps and this will also be difficult if you have visitors. Setting visiting times for friends and relatives will allow you to plan your day and get the rest you need.

Midwife Visits

Your midwife will visit the day after you go home but, depending on how straightforward your birth was, it might be six days until she calls again. At this day 6 visit she will discuss the 'Heel Spot Test' and if you consent to this it will be carried out during that visit. The 'Heel Spot Test' is carried out to test for a number of conditions that can either be treated with medication or diet. For more information on this screening test you can visit the 'NHS choices' website.

Your midwife will also provide you with a contact number to request additional visits and support if you have feeding problems or any other concerns. The change in the frequency of visits was introduced to ensure that women who needed extra support were able to have this. For some women especially those with more than one child they do not need the same amount of visits as women with their first baby. When you are receiving visits every day it requires you to be at home for a large proportion of that day which may be inconvenient, especially if you did not need a visit. This allows you more flexibility and access to assistance when you need it rather than a generalised plan of care, but you need to request that assistance. If your partner feels that you, or he, need some help he can also contact your community midwife and request a visit.

Help at Home

Your partner will need to do most of the daily running of your home for the first few weeks. As you fall into a routine your sole responsibility will be feeding your baby, so cleaning ironing and cooking can wait. If your partner can organise the cleaning, washing and ironing to be done that will leave only the cooking. If you have had time before your birth you may have been able to prepare and freeze meals in advance, if not ask friends and family to help. It is only for a few weeks and this extra help will allow you stress free time to establish your breastfeeding and bond with your baby.

If you are formula feeding then others can do that. Again, you need to listen to your body as rest will be just as important for you. Even if your partner is helping with night feeds you will still have a broken sleep pattern and it is important that you are able to catch up with this. As you are not breastfeeding your body will not be producing the same volume and type of hormones that aid a deeper, more restful sleep.

Out and About, Breastfeeding

For a simple trip to the shops or afternoon outing all you will need is the following if you are breastfeeding:

- Nappies, one for every two hours you will be out
- Cotton wool or baby wipes
- Bib
- One change of clothes
- Muslin
- Large scarf or pashmina

Take a changing mat if you wish, however a piece of muslin is just as effective and is less roomy. You will not need a changing bag if your handbag is big enough. The large scarf can be worn and used to cover your breasts while you are latching him on as this can be tricky at first and breastfeeding bras and breast pads are a must. Shirts or blouses are the easiest clothes for breastfeeding and as your baby establishes his feeding you will find that he will find your nipple himself and will need only slight prompting to attach.

Out and About, Formula Feeding

Formula feeding mothers have it harder as more equipment is needed. Current guidance on formula feeds is that they are made up as needed and not in advance. This means taking either cartons of your formula or bottles made up with water and separate tubs of measured powder. In addition to this you will need:

- Nappies, one for every two hours you will be out
- Cotton wool or baby wipes
- Bibs
- Muslin
- Bottles and powder or cartons, enough for each feed plus one extra for emergencies
- One change of clothes

If your baby prefers warm milk a flask of hot water to heat his milk needs to be included too. Unless you use an enormous handbag it is likely you will need to take a changing bag. When buying a changing bag spare a thought for your partner, who will probably also carry it, so it's best to avoid extremely feminine styles.

The first time you head out with your newborn you will undoubtedly be nervous. Take a friend or family member with you that first time, preferably one who has experience with babies. Try taking him to a family friendly area first and if you are offered help by other parents accept it, don't be embarrassed, they too have been there and understand. The most difficult time will be when he starts to cry. Despite knowing he's crying because he is hungry you will still feel slightly anxious. Try to relax, babies cry and everyone around you will understand this. They will not judge even though you may think they do. After a few hours you will relax into it and enjoy it and after a few days you'll wonder why you were ever worried.

Worries and Concerns

After any birth, but especially your first, you will undoubtedly have concerns. You might be concerned for your baby or yourself, but it is important that you act upon those concerns. There really is such a thing as a mother's instinct, so if you are concerned at all about your baby ask you G.P. or midwife to visit. If after they have visited you still feel concerned or you feel they have not listened you should take you baby to your local emergency department. You will be reassured that there is nothing wrong or if a problem is found then you will have been justified in your anxiety.

Occasionally you will worry about yourself. You may have problems going to the toilet or you may have emotional worries. You would normally inform your midwife or G.P. if you suffer with physical problems and the same applies to your psychological wellbeing. There is no need to worry that they will judge you in any way. You should be enjoying this time with your baby and the sooner you can get help the quicker you will be able to enjoy him properly.

Birth Afterthoughts

Maybe you had the birth you wanted and you were shown compassion and kindness whilst in labour. For the majority of women this is how childbirth will be. But a minority will look back at the birth with anger, sadness and possibly trauma. The birth might have been traumatic for you, despite the views of those around you. Just as many women who had a quick trouble-free labour are traumatised when compared to those who had an assisted labour and felt empowered. Much of your feelings are down to the perceived care you experienced during pregnancy and birth. Those who feel empowered are usually those who were prepared for an assisted birth and were cared for in a respectful and dignified manner allowing them control over their birth.

You can voice your feelings to the labour ward manager and ask for a meeting to review your birth. They will arrange for a midwife, obstetrician, or both, to go through your birth with you and answer all of your questions. They will make plans for your care in pregnancy, labour and birth should you wish to have another baby.

If you want to complain about the care you received your first contact should be the Head of Midwifery at your local hospital. Their contact information should be available on the hospital's website.

Weeks or months after a birth debrief following an emergency, such as shoulder dystocia or postpartum haemorrhage, you may have many unanswered questions. You can either contact your consultant obstetrician's secretary for an appointment or again the labour ward manager or Head of Midwifery. Each of these points of contact will be able to arrange a meeting to discuss your concerns. During that meeting you should take with you a list of all the questions you wish to ask and also your partner or a friend to offer support. Those providing this session will be open and honest with you and this should help you come to terms with your birth experience.

Baby Blues

After a few days at home with your newborn you will begin to understand his routine and be able to anticipate when he will sleep and need feeding. After a few days you may become tearful and anxious and be overwhelmed by trivial matters. These emotions are a normal part of the transition to motherhood. It is known as the 'baby blues' and affects around eight out of ten women. The blues usually fade in a few weeks and the simplest and quickest way to resolve them is to treat the cause.

You will be sleep deprived, anxious over his wellbeing, being flooded by hormones and most likely attempting to be 'Supermum'. You will probably still be doing most of the housework you did before the birth and no matter how many times you are told to slow down and rest you will not listen. If you will not listen to your family, then listen to your body which is telling you to rest.

Midwives struggle to enforce rest on women and don't wish to interfere by telling partners they need to relax. Pregnancy and childbirth are natural, not an illness, however motherhood, breastfeeding and sleep deprivation will take their toll if you do not get enough nourishment, fluids and rest. Conceding that you cannot do it all is difficult, but here's what you need to do:

- Run a bath – Your partner can take your baby to you if he needs to be fed.
- Order a takeaway for dinner that night.
- Tell your partner that the washing, ironing and cooking for the next week will need to be done by him or be organised by friends of family.
- Once you have had dinner and your baby has had his evening feed, go to bed.
- Your partner needs to reassure you that your baby is fine and you are doing a brilliant job.
- Accept the compliments and the fact that you feel like this.

By doing this you are not admitting defeat, you are treating the physical and psychological impact of sleep deprivation and exhaustion and the symptoms of baby blues.

Postnatal Depression

This is not 'baby blues' in that it will not pass after a few days. The symptoms of postnatal depression can persist for months and for some, if left untreated, can become a long-term problem. Postnatal depression can begin to develop in the first four to six weeks after childbirth, however some women may not develop symptoms for months later. The usual symptoms are:

- Symptoms of the baby blues that persist longer than expected.
- Persistent feelings of sadness and low mood
- Difficulty falling asleep
- Loss of interest in the world around you
- No longer enjoying the things you used to
- Feeling tired all the time
- Feelings of guilt or self-blame
- Poor or increased appetite
- Crying for no reason
- Lack of personal hygiene
- Withdrawing from friends and family
- Worried there is something wrong with your baby

The condition can interfere with daily life and the way you care for your baby. You might feel incapable of looking after him, or scared to leave your house to meet friends

It is common to have thoughts about harming your baby. At this point most women will seek advice. Your family will normally notice the condition before you do and they may ask you to seek help from your G.P. Some may even contact them on your behalf. Once contact has been made and you have opened up and received treatment you can begin to get well again as postnatal depression needs proper treatment, you will not just snap out of it.

It is important to remember you are not being punished for anything and you are most definitely not a bad mother. There is no rhyme or reason why *you* should suffer from postnatal depression. Given time and treatment you will get back to the way you were and the mother you want to be. You will enjoy spending time with him without always feeling anxious and you will have the energy to look after your family.

Chapter 19

Taking care of Baby & You

Breastfeeding

Be prepared! Babies cry, and sometimes they really will cry for no reason at all. You will have fed them, changed them and cuddled them, yet nothing seems to have made a difference. Some parents are lucky in that their baby settles easily and cries very little while other parents find their babies cry most of the time. This only last a short time but if you are breastfeeding you might conclude that it is your milk that is causing the problem; but you mustn't, it is extremely unlikely you will not produce the correct quantity or quality of milk.

Well-meaning friends and family might advise you to give your baby a bottle. If there is nothing wrong with your milk supply, which there will not be, then this will achieve nothing. A breastfed baby does not cry more than a formula fed baby, they just feed more often.

A few reassurances that he is feeding well and receiving adequate amounts:

- He will feed eight times or more in 24 hours.
- He will feed for five to 45 minutes per feed.
- He will take himself off your breast when he is finished.

- His skin colour is normal although slight jaundice is also common.
- He is calm and relaxed during feeds and content afterwards.

If he is not meeting these criteria you should inform your midwife and ask her to visit. He should also have the following wet and dirty nappies for the corresponding days:

Wet Nappies

Day 1 and 2	1 or 2 in 24 hours
Day 3 and 4	3 or more in 24 hours
Day 5 and 6	5 or more in 24 hours, wet and as heavy as 3 tablespoons of water.
Day 7 – 28	6 or more wet and heavy as above.

Dirty Nappies

Day 1 and 2	1 or more in 24 hours, black and tar like .
Day 3 and 4	2 or more, changing in colour (brown/green/yellow) and now looser.
Day 5 and 6	2 or more yellow, slightly watery
Day 7 – 28	2 or more and at least the size of a £2 coin and now with a 'mustard seed' appearance.

If he does not meet these criteria you should contact your midwife and request a visit. Providing that your baby's nappies correspond with this and he is gaining weight then your milk supply is adequate.

A few tips to stop his crying - you need to start with the basics first:

- Change his nappy.
- Give him a cuddle.
- Try feeding him again, he may be cluster feeding.
- Give him a bath or take him out in the car.

It might seem he is crying all the time but it is more likely that he cries when not being fed or not being held. If this is the case don't worry about cuddling him or having him with you, your instinct as a mother will guide you.

If he is struggling to settle, even when feeding, or if your breasts are painful, then it is time to contact your midwife and request a visit. It is most likely a problem with his positioning on your breast. You should also contact your midwife if you are worried about your baby's colour, for example if he appears yellow, always falls asleep on the breast or never finishes the feed himself. Some pointers from your midwife should sort this out. If you become concerned about him in the middle of the night then contact your labour ward for advice, they will be more than happy to help.

Care Following a Caesarean Section

If you gave birth by Caesarean section then you really will need to take it slowly and take care of your recovering body and wound. There are several layers of sutures in your lower abdomen and you have undergone major abdominal surgery. You will experience pain and should have been provided with pain relief to take home. Most women mistakenly fail to take pain relief regularly and the more pain you have, the less mobile and active you will be, and paradoxically less mobility leads to more pain.

Although you will be encouraged to be mobile you will still need to rest when required. You need to avoid activity that strains your stomach muscles; this includes standing for prolonged periods, carrying heavy bags and housework. You should avoid lifting anything other than your baby for six weeks. You should receive advice from your obstetrician on when it will be safe to drive again; usually around four to six weeks following surgery or when you can perform an emergency stop without any undue pain. You need to inform your insurance company beforehand.

Breastfeeding mums will have been given medication that will not affect their milk. If you are given medication that cannot be taken whilst breastfeeding you will be expressly informed of this. Medication will have dosage instructions to ensure you are comfortable and pain free at rest and pain relief is far more effective if you stay on top of it.

Some women have a higher pain tolerance and paracetamol is adequate for this group of women. Others have a lower pain threshold and might need additional drugs.

If you do have any concerns, or suffer from any of the following then you should contact your midwife for advice:

- If you feel hot, unwell or have flu-like symptoms.
- If you notice a smelly discharge from your vagina.
- If your bleeding becomes heavier.
- If the pain in your abdomen increases.
- If the pain around your wound increases.
- If you notice discharge from your wound
- If the area around your wound becomes red or hot.

There are many reasons why symptoms occur but your midwife will usually first check for infection. Swabs from your vagina and wound will be taken and the test results known in a few days. You midwife might ask your G.P. to visit if she is concerned you might need antibiotics before the results are back.

The obstetrician can use staples, absorbable suture maternal or non-absorbable sutures to close your wound. If they not absorbable they will be removed by your community midwife. The date they need removing will be on your hospital discharge information. Wound dressings stay on for a week and are therefore waterproof.

Hygiene following any contractions is vital and you should bathe every day. After your dressing is removed ensure the wound is dried thoroughly and change your sanitary pads at least every four hours. Should you or your partner have any concerns, contact your labour ward for advice.

Taking Care of Your Perineum

Up to eight women out of ten receive some kind of cut or tear to their vagina or labia and advice on how to care for these tears and pain relief is given in hospital. The discomfort is mostly from swelling to the tissues of your vagina, labia and perineum and the most effective treatment is ice. You can buy specialist gel packs for your perineal area or, providing they are clean anything frozen will do. You need to apply a sterile gauze swab over the ice pack and then apply it to your perineum for ten minutes.

Healing tissue requires an adequate blood supply. Applying ice reduces blood supply around the area and with it the fluid that causes the swelling. Because of this reduction in blood supply the use of an ice pack is advised for only two days. Pain killers will also prevent discomfort, but it may take three weeks before you can sit down properly without pain relief. Whilst recovering you will find it most comfortable to sit on one or other bottom cheek and pillows or cushions will help with this.

Midwives no longer routinely check your perineum because the majority of women experience no problems as they heal. Some women notice the pain in their perineum becomes worse. If you complain of any of the following you should contact your community midwife and request a visit:

- Pain in your perineum that is becoming worse rather than better.
- Discharge from your perineal wound.
- If the area feels hot and tender.
- If the wound appears to be open.
- Smelly discharge from your vagina.
- Increased blood loss.
- Feeling hot, unwell or have flu like symptoms.

The wound needs to be kept clean and dry. Bathe regularly, dry it thoroughly and change your pads at least every four hours. Your lochia (the normal blood stained discharge) will continue for around three weeks, becoming gradually lighter in colour before stopping completely. Over exertion or more frequent breast feeds can increase this blood loss and you should always contact your midwife for advice on any matter that concerns you.

Pelvic Floor Exercises

Pelvic floor exercises are extremely important and you can begin them as soon as you like after the birth, providing you do not have a catheter sited.

Your pelvic floor has been stretched during pregnancy and birth. Its role is vital in supporting the organs in your pelvis. If it becomes weak its ability to support the bladder, urethra, intestines and uterus is compromised and can lead to urinary and faecal incontinence and prolapse. Women who have had three or more children or given birth to heavier babies tend to weaker pelvic floor.

Performing simple exercises strengthens the muscle. Decide on a trigger to remind you to do the exercises, perhaps each time you have a meal. Ideally you should exercise three times per day but you may need to work up to this.

Sit comfortably and without clenching your buttocks or stomach muscles try to clench the muscle around your urethra (the tube you pass urine from). Some women find it easier to imagine that they are trying to prevent themselves from passing urine. Next, squeeze your vagina and then the muscles around your back passage, as if preventing wind from escaping but remember not to clench your buttocks. Once you have the muscles tightened around them lift them upwards as you tighten. Try to hold this for up to ten seconds and then relax.

Repeat this ten times. As your pelvic floor strengthens you will be able to hold the squeeze longer and do them more frequently. You will notice the results after a few months, including a greater sensitivity during sexual intercourse. You should continue these exercises even when you feel that they have worked as it will keep the pelvic floor strong.

It is important that you do not strain when you go to the toilet. When you open your bowels place a wad of toilet paper in front of your back passage and press firmly, this should make it more comfortable. Drinking one to three litres of fluid a day also helps and breastfeeding mums may need more and you should drink to thirst.

Diet and Exercise

You will gradually lose the weight that you gained during pregnancy after the birth. Breastfeeding helps in this, as does sensible eating and gentle exercise. It is vital you eat well as your body recovers from pregnancy and childbirth. It is important not to diet as your body will naturally lose the weight through moderate changes to your portion size and healthier choices.

If breastfeeding you will need approximately 2,500 calories per day rather than the usual 2,000 calories. The extra calories go to the nutrients your baby receives. Once you have stopped breastfeeding you will be able to be stricter with your calorie intake.

If formula feeding wait at least two months after giving birth before dieting and make sure the diet is sustainable, such as a calorie controlled diet.

Exercise is great for weight loss after birth. You normally have a check-up with your G.P. after eight weeks and they will advise you whether it is safe to exercise strenuously. Initial exercises should be gentle, such as walking or yoga.

Gradually build the level of exercise over a period of two to six months. After six months you should be able to perform any exercise you wish, providing that you are fit enough of course.

If you are recovering from a Caesarean section you will usually be advised to wait for twelve weeks after the operation before starting strenuous exercise. However, gentle exercise is allowed earlier. If you enjoyed running before childbirth you should wait six months until resuming - longer if you are breastfeeding to prevent back and pelvic floor problems.

If in doubt speak to a specialist personal trainer in postnatal exercise, better still join a postnatal exercise class where you can exercise in groups with your baby, and meet new friends.

'What Did We Do Before He Came Along?'

As you move on from your birth experience you will gradually begin to feel like yourself again. Your sleep patterns will begin to return to normal and your body will feel as strong as it once did. Now is the time to pay attention to your relationship and each other. Make time for yourselves together and separately and pamper yourself if you feel you need it, you deserve it, you have both achieved something truly amazing.

This journey that began so many months ago is not at an end but merely at the beginning of an enlightening and inspiring period of your lives. Your labour itself is just a small bump on that road and whichever methods you use to manage your labour and whichever way you choose to give birth will not and should not define you both as parents. What will define you is the love and support you give each other and your

child. You will forever ask each other that immortal question;
'*What did we do with our time before he came along?*'

Active Birth Centre

Information on reclaiming your body and birth rite
www.activebirthcentre.com

A.I.M.S. (Association for Improvements in Maternity Services)

They will point you in the right direction if you are having difficulty with your care providers in achieving the care and birth of your choice.
www.aims.org.uk

Bespoke Birthing Midwifery Practice

Independent Midwifery practice based in Yorkshire.
www.bespokebirthing.co.uk

Birth Choice UK

Provides detailed birth outcome data on hospitals and maternity care in the U.K., allowing you to decide on your place of birth.
www.birthchoiceuk.com

Birth Trauma Association

A charity offering support to women who have had a traumatic birth experience.
www.birthtraumaassociation.org.uk

The Breastfeeding Network

An independent source of source and information for breastfeeding

www.breastfeeding.co.uk

Caesarean Birth Information

For up to date information regarding your choices for caesarean sections and VBAC

www.caesarean.org.uk

Doula UK

For information and help with finding a doula in your area

www.doula.org.uk

Dr Foster Hospital Guide

Gives guidance on hospital safety figures

www.drfosterhealth.co.uk

Group B Strep Support Group

Provides information, support and research on Group B Streptococcus

www.gbss.org.uk

Home Birth

For up to date information on homebirths and how to arrange one

www.homebirth.org.uk

Independent Midwives U.K.

For up to date advice and information on independent midwives, pregnancy, labour and birth.
www.independentmidwives.org.uk

Mind

An organisation that provides support to women with postnatal depression
www.mind.org.uk

N.C.T. (National Childbirth Trust)

An organisation that provides birth and breastfeeding education, support and organises sales for parents to be
www.nct.org.uk

National Institute for Clinical Excellence (NICE)

Guidance for professionals and public
www.nice.org.uk

Royal College of Obstetricians and Gynaecologists (RCOG)

Provides information to professionals and the public on care in pregnancy, labour and the postnatal period
www.rcog.org.uk

Slimming World

Support with healthy eating and limiting weight gain in pregnancy and whilst breastfeeding www.slimmingworld.com

Twins and Multiple Birth Association - (Tamba)
Offering advice and support to parents with multiple births
www.tamba.org.uk

Water birth International
Informative articles about the advantages of birth in water
www.waterbirth .org

References

ASSISTED BIRTHS

Royal College of Obstetricians and Gynaecologists
http://www.rcog.org.uk/files/rcog-
corp/An%20Assisted%20Vaginal%20Birth_0.pdf

BIRTHPLACE STUDY

Hollowell J, Puddicombe D, Rowe R, Linsell L, Hardy P, Stewart M, et al 2011. The Birthplace national prospective cohort study: perinatal and maternal outcomes by planned place of birth. Birthplace in England research programme. *British Medical Journal, 343, 7400.*

BREECH BABIES

Hannah ME, Hannah WJ, Hewson SA, Hodnett ED, Saigal S, Willan AR. 2000, Planned caesarean section versus planned vaginal birth for breech presentation at term: a randomised multicentre trial. Term Breech Trial Collaborative Group. *Lancet.* Oct 21;356(9239):1375-83.

CAESAREAN SECTION

CG132 Caesarean Section – *National Institute for Health and Clinical   Excellence*, www.nice.org.uk/nicemedia/live/13620/57166/57166.pdf

MacKenzie IZ, Cooke I; What is a reasonable time from decision-to-delivery by caesarean section? Evidence from 415 deliveries. *British Journal of Obstetrics and Gynaecology.* 2002 May;109(5):498-504.

DELAYED CORD CLAMPING

Andersson O, Hellström-Westas L, Andersson J, Domellöf,, 2011. Effect of delayed versus early umbilical cord clamping on neonatal outcomes and iron status at 4 months: a randomised controlled trial. *British Medical Journal;343:d7157*

EPISIOTOMY

Carroli G, Belizan J. Episiotomy for vaginal birth. *Cochrane Database of Systematic Reviews* 2007, Issue 4. Art. No.: CD000081. DOI: 10.1002/14651858.CD000081.

GROUP B STREPTOCOCCUS

GBSS Medical Panel 2012, Streptococcus B in pregnancy: to screen or not to screen? *British Medical Journal,* April.

Daniels JP, Gray J, Pattison HM 2011, Intrapartum tests for group B streptococcus: accuracy and acceptability of screening, *British Journal of Obstetrics and Gynaecology* Jan, 118(2), 257 – 65

Gray R, Hills RK, Khan KS; GBS Collaborative Group. *British Journal of Obstetrics and Gynaecology.* 2011 Jan;118(2):257-65.

Heath PT, Balfour G, Tighe H, Verlander NQ, Lamagni T, Efstratiou A. 2009 Group B streptococcal disease in infants: a case control study. May. *Arch Dis Child.*

MONITORING BABY'S HEART RATE

Wiberg-Itzel E, Lipponer C, Norman M, et al; Determination of pH or lactate in fetal scalp blood in management of intrapartum fetal distress: randomised controlled multicentre trial. *British Medical Journal.* 2008 Jun 7;336(7656):1284-7. Epub 2008 May 25.

Alfirevic Z, Devane D, Gyte GM; Continuous cardiotocography (CTG) as a form of electronic fetal monitoring (EFM) for fetal assessment during labour. *Cochrane Database Systematic Review.* 2006 Jul 19;3:CD006066.

PERINEAL MASSAGE

Beckmann MM, Garrett AJ; Antenatal perineal massage for reducing perineal trauma. *Cochrane Database Systematic Review.* 2006 Jan 25;(1):CD005123.

Stamp G, Kruzins G, Crowther C; Perineal massage in labour and prevention of perineal trauma: randomised controlled trial. *British Medical Journal.* 2001 May 26;322(7297):1277-80

PERINEAL SUTURING

Fleming VE, Hagen S, Niven C; Does perineal suturing make a difference? The SUNS trial. *British journal of Obstetrics and Gynaecology.* 2003 Jul;110(7):684-9.

Leeman LM, Rogers RG, Greulich B, et al; Do unsutured second-degree perineal lacerations affect postpartum functional outcomes? *Journal of the American Board of Family Medicine*. 2007 Sep-Oct;20(5):451-7.

Sleep J, Grant A, Garcia J, et al; West Berkshire perineal management trial. *British Medical Journal* (Clin Res Ed). 1984 Sep 8;289(6445):587-90.

PERINEUM

McCandlish R, Bowler U, van Asten H, Berridge G, Winter C, Sames L, et al. A randomised controlled trial of care of the perineum during the second stage of normal labour. *British Journal of Obstetrics and Gynaecology*. 1998;105:1262–1272.

PRELABOUR RUPTURE OF MEMBRANES

http://www.nice.org.uk/nicemedia/pdf/IPCNICEGuidance.pdf page 39 - 41.

THIRD STAGE OF LABOUR

McDonald SJ, Abbott JM, Higgins SP, 2009. Prophylactic ergometrine-oxytocin versus oxytocin for the third stage of labour. *Cochrane Database Systematic Review*. Published Online: April 15, 2009.

Prendiville W, Harding J, Elbourne D, Stirrat G., 1988 The Bristol third stage trial: active versus physiological management of the third stage of labour. *British Medical Journal*; 297:1295–300.

Rogers J, Wood J, McCandlish R, Ayers S, Truesdale A, Elbourne D,1998. Active versus expectant management of third stage of labour: the Hinchingbrooke randomised controlled trial. *Lancet*. Mar 7;351(9104):693-9.

TWIN PREGNANCY AND INDUCTION OF LABOUR

Dodd J, Crowther C, Haslam R, Robinson J. 2012 Elective birth at 37 weeks of gestation versus standard care for women with an uncomplicated twin pregnancy at term: the Twins Timing of Birth Randomised Trial. *British Journal of Obstetrics & Gyneacology*;119:964–974.

VITAMIN K FOR BABIES

Neonatal Vitamin K – *National institute of clinical Excellence*, Routine postnatal care of women and their babies, http://www.nice.org.uk/nicemedia/pdf/CG37NICEguideline.pdf

Busfield A, Samuel R, McNinch A, Tripp J, 2011. Vitamin K Deficiency Bleeding after NICE guidance and withdrawal of Konakion Neonatal: British Paediatric Surveillance Unit study, 2006–2008 *Arch Dis Child* ;**98**:41-47 doi:10.1136/archdischild-2011-301029

Acknowledgements

The literary embers of this book have burned in my head for many years. I had so much I wanted to say but just never got around to putting them on paper, until now. There are so many people who helped with the writing of this book and none more so than my husband who, in his own words, was a single parent for many months. To my beautiful children Francesca and Ruairidh for selflessly doing without their mummy for many months and being so understanding for people so young. To my wonderful sister Morvern, for the hours she spent toiling with the first draft of this manuscript and giving advice on tailoring it for women. To my mother Beeshie, another midwife, for all her support, persuasion and persistence in writing this book. To my friend Brighdin who unwittingly gave me the inspiration to turn a few pages of information into this book. To another Lesley, an inspirational doula whose insight helped mould this book into what you see now. To the midwives who taught me this art (and still do) and to all my colleagues who still inspire me. And finally to the women I have had the privilege to meet and care for in my career as a midwife you have taught me so much and humbled me greatly along the way, thank you.

About the Author

Lesley grew up in a small town in Scotland on the beautiful peninsula of Kintyre. She began her nursing career in Glasgow in 1997 and moved to Newcastle in 2000 where, in 2001 she began her midwifery training. Lesley worked in Newcastle's Royal Victoria Infirmary from 2003 – 2006 where she worked primarily on delivery suite and undertook research into the second stage of labour. She then left Newcastle for Leeds in 2006 where she worked with Leeds Teaching Hospitals NHS Trust in both delivery suite and in the community as a community midwife, gaining qualifications in advanced practice and also appearing on Channel 4's 'One born Every Minute'. In 2013 she began studying for a Master's degree in Clinical Research Methods with the University of Leeds.

.... Whilst studying, Lesley set up 'Bespoke Birthing Midwifery Practice' offering tailored, private midwifery care for all aspects of pregnancy, birth and baby in addition to birth education and hypnobirthing. She currently practises as an independent midwife in Yorkshire, with her business going from strength to strength.